Praise for Approaching Sunris

Everyone has a story and each one is important. Joanne's story is not just pertinent, it's urgent! Cancer is no one's friend and, like a thief, stole my best friend in 2012. Our health is our greatest asset and when cancer looms we can't help but be overwhelmed with feelings of anxiety, insecurity and doubt. Beyond medicine, the strongest ally is someone who's lived it, heard the diagnosis, faced their own mortality and is not simply surviving, but thriving. This uplifting biography is literary caffeine with no side effects. The intellectual unveiling of this beautiful soul has the power to encourage and inspire anyone. Share it with a friend, you may change the trajectory of their life and your own! - **Michael "Pinball" Clemons.**

Joanne Stacey is one of the most positive people I have ever met. She embraced her breast cancer experience with hope and trust in her health-care team and now commits her energy and caring to helping others through her story. Tenacious, positive about life and with a generous heart and spirit, Joanne continues to be a force for good. Her willingness to share a myriad of helpful advice with individuals and their support network certainly buffers the realities of a cancer journey. – **Pearl F. Veenema. FAHP, President and CEO, Hamilton Health Sciences Foundation.**

I have come to know Joanne as someone who is governed by servitude, and truly wants to use her own devastating cancer diagnosis, ensuing treatment and all it entails, to better the lives of others. I commend this remarkable cancer survivor on sharing her story, as it is profoundly important for others. While there is ample scientific and methodical information about cancer, and you can Google anything these days, it's quite often the personal stories and experiences that patients and their families are truly looking for. It's the little nuggets of information and tricks of getting by in their day-to-day lives that end up making the most impact. Through this book, and her life, Joanne has offered another voice in the dialogue of cancer, and has truly become an inspiration to those who know her and read her story. – **Marie Goldwater, Journalist**

Joanne's manuscript was sent to me this week, and I have to say this is a powerful, and very useful, read. Anyone that has been diagnosed with breast cancer should read this book: Joanne is the bravest woman I know and the way she handled her disease was nothing less than heroic. God bless her, and all who have this battle ahead of them - Joanne with help get you through this. -**Jo-Ann Porter, Owner, Exquisite Wines.**

This book is dedicated to helping people face their personal crises. Joanne is a survivor; she not only faced the challenges of cancer, she won. She is continuing to share her stories for others, to give them Hope, Faith, and Perseverance. She shows how to fight the "good fight" and the importance of trusting your family, friends and medical team in your own personal battles. Like the football players, "The Young Thundering Herd" at Marshall University, she is a Winner and a Giver. - **Jack Lengyel, Head Football Coach, Marshall University (Retired), "WE ARE Marshall."**

To anyone who has been diagnosed with breast cancer, Joanne Stacey, a former patient and now friend of mine, has woven her story into an engaging biography, making a gift of her very personal and intimate experience. This book gives a synopsis of the Journey through diagnosis to survivorship! The tale is heartwarming and inclusive of health care providers, family, and friends and speaks to the many roller-coaster emotions that each experiences. This book demonstrates what one positive patient survivor can accomplish and how this energy and experience can benefit others who will embark on this cancer journey! I thoroughly enjoyed reading this personal story of courage and survivorship! - **Kathy Coskey RN BSCN CCRP Con(c)**

This book is raw with strength, courage & love. It brings comfort to know that we are not alone in this journey and that anything is possible and that cancer doesn't mean the worst. It's full of knowledge and tools that shed light on treatment and recovery. Wonderful read!! - **Laura Pflug Region Coordinator, Investors Group Financial Services Inc.**

Approaching Sunrise

My Personal Journey with Breast Cancer
from Diagnosis to Survival

Joanne Stacey

Edited by: Darrin Griffiths, Ed.D.
Copy Edited by: Steve Viau

Cover Design: Emily Rucker
Interior Design: Jim Bisakowski - bookdesign.ca

978-0-9918626-7-2

DEDICATION

Dedicated to my Mom, a very gentle, kind, simple spirit full of passion and always generous. She showed a compassion and sensitivity to everyone, especially the underdogs and the animals. Mom, you have shown me a patience and a courage the past few months that I had not seen so strongly in you before. Thank you for letting me be a little more outgoing or aggressive in my ways, as you were unsure sometimes of my manner. You shared your philanthropic ways and beliefs with me and showed me how not to sweat the small stuff!

As said in the film ONE TRUE THING with Meryl Streep, one of my Mom's and my favourite actresses,

"Terminal Illness is a thief robbing you of someone you love. It is also a teacher – it teaches you about death, sacrifice, love, hope, grief, honour and dignity. But mostly it teaches you about the value of living your life with joy each and every single day you can."

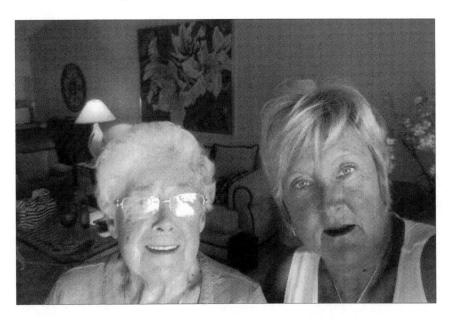

CONTENTS

Foreword

In my role as a Regional Director with Investors Group, Canada's largest and oldest comprehensive financial planning company, I have the privilege of leading a dedicated group of men and women committed to helping as many families as possible achieve both financial independence and financial security. Providing for – and protecting against – all of life's inevitabilities represents the principal foundation of all our work.

It goes without saying, therefore, that the reality of our chosen profession is that far too often we witness far too many clients become sick. All of us it seems have been specifically touched by cancer. The feeling that permeates when cancer strikes someone you know and love is incomprehensible. It's incredibly difficult to articulate in words how my family and I felt when Joanne Stacey informed us that she was diagnosed with breast cancer. At the time, Joanne was serving as my Executive Assistant, but our relationship existed on a much more profound and significant level. Joanne, her husband Bob and their children were an extension of my own family. My wife Janice and I were – and are – genuinely blessed and fortunate to have the Stacey family in our lives.

In my mind, Joanne has always been defined by her boundless energy, her zest for life, her love of family and passion for her community. I'm convinced that success in life is the result of embracing every situation with the "right" attitude. Joanne's attitude and enthusiasm is infectious. This is why cancer had no chance.

Joanne has decided to courageously document her journey; to offer inspiration and hope to others. Joanne has demonstrated most importantly that a cancer diagnosis is not a death sentence. Her personal experience has created an overwhelming desire to educate other women facing similar circumstances. To make a difference. Beating cancer requires an assault on many fronts. We are all acutely aware of the medical advancements regarding the treatment of breast cancer. Never underestimate, however, the power of your mind and the influence of positive thinking. Joanne's mental approach was her greatest asset and the greatest gift she can share in her story to empower others.

Joanne's vibration, her invisible aura of positivity, refused to wane after her diagnosis. I would argue that it became even more intense. In no way would she permit cancer to defeat her, to deny her the ability to watch her children and grandchildren grow to live happy, healthy and productive lives. She refused to feel sorry for herself and her unconditional belief in herself and her determination to beat this dreaded disease was non-negotiable. Given this motivation it was only natural that all of us – friends, family and colleagues alike – would willingly and collectively rally around her with abundant love and provide whatever support was required in her battle. A battle not surprisingly that proved victorious. Again, cancer had no chance.

The Apostle Mark once said that anyone who wishes to be great must be a servant to all and put themselves last. In both my personal and professional life rarely have I met anyone who embodies these words more than Joanne Stacey. This book is a summation of a life dedicated to helping and educating others. It is, and always has been, an honour for me to be associated with this incredible human being.

Jon Jurus, Regional Director, Investors Group

Jon has been a very special man and coach in my life. As his executive assistant and event coordinator over 25 years, we worked closely together and became very close. He shares much with my husband as they were both University football players and amazing coaches on and off the field. Jon is a true coach and mentor and has always lead by example in his professional and personal life. This man has enriched my life in so many ways; he taught me some of the most significant life lessons and has always been there for me. He may be the Regional Director of a successful financial office, but he is more a simple man with a huge heart and always puts his family, friends and staff first.

INTRODUCTION

I had not completed my book—life continued to get in the way and there just wasn't the time to try to get it more organized. I needed good quiet uninterrupted time! But after my most recent hospital stay and seeing my Mom become older and more confused with dementia after suffering a stroke, I thought it was time to consider completing it.

My Mom would like to reread my story and share in its life because she was a big part of this book. My Mom Joan was diagnosed with Breast Cancer in the spring of 2006 and required a lumpectomy and radiation. She was my first personal, close connection to cancer. Her initial diagnosis began as a social outing to the United States. My mom was unable to have an immediate MRI in our region of Halton (Ontario), so she was given a requisition from a GP here to have one done over the border at a clinic.

We decided to make a family weekend of it to eat out, shop and share a hotel. We always have good laughs on our cross border shopping trips, but this adventure started sooner. While going through Customs, the officers there pulled us over to make sure that our reason for visiting the United States was valid. They had to search us. Mom thought this was comical. We had a female customs clerk pat us down to ensure our story was accurate, and that we did not pose a security risk. I even had the requisition for the clinic in Buffalo to show to the custom's official and eventually we were cleared for entry to the United States.

This was winter, and it was cold, so we didn't walk too far and had dinner in the hotel across the road from the clinic. The MRI would be of the breast. We did not want to wait months in our community but by crossing the border we could pay in US currency to have the testing done and get results immediately. It was a very frustrating process because I thought our medical system was pretty good compared to the one in the United States.

We enjoyed the weekend and spoke little of the test. As I saw things, Mom has always been healthy and we all believed that any results would be nothing too exciting. At the same time, we were also relieved that we would soon know the outcome.

I say this is my first personal experience with cancer involving a significant person close to me. I have had acquaintances die from the disease (as well as the parents of friends like anyone else). However, I hadn't felt I had been hit heavily yet by cancer.

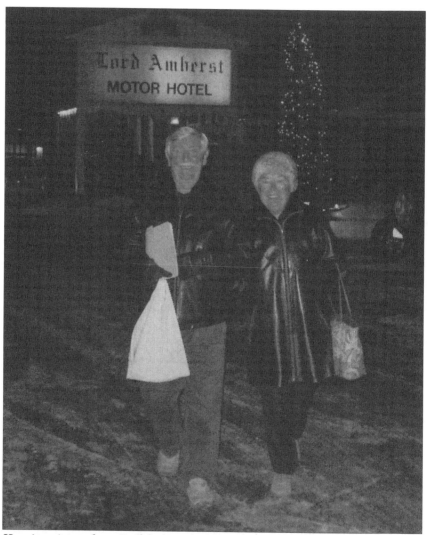

Here is a picture from Buffalo (2005) when mom, dad, and I went for mom's MRI for a breast lump.

My Mom's results were more frightening than we had anticipated. We learned that she had breast cancer, and that she would proceed with discussions and a treatment plan. Mom and Dad said little of the cancer and downplayed it; they shared little because they are fairly private and did not want to worry us.

They saw an oncologist at Credit Valley and Mom chose a lumpectomy. My dad and I picked my Mom up after an outpatient surgery. She appeared to be in good spirits but she was also tired and wanted to return home to sleep. Mom was uncomfortable from the bandages and drain; Dad and I just did what we could to make her feel more comfortable. At the time, Mom was 72 and had been very healthy. She was an active curler, bridge player and participated in her sorority and various community organizations. I didn't ask too many questions about her experiences during the outpatient surgery or get too involved.

My parents didn't volunteer a lot about the process, but they seemed happy with the choice she made. They were very pleased with their surgeon, and that the radiation treatment that would start soon. I believed it to be a small tumor because it only required a lumpectomy and radiation, without any rounds of chemotherapy.

I took Mom to radiation a few times and it was a social event for her. She and Dad really enjoyed the staff at the Juravinski Cancer Centre and couldn't say enough positive things of the care she received.

I took her flowers on the last day of her treatment and she was distributing "Thank You" cards to the staff who took care of her over the 6-8 weeks of radiation. This treatment never appeared to disrupt any of my parents' plans or travel. Dad was happy to get Mom to most of her treatments and would always pick up her medications, as well as the prosthesis she needed as a piece to fit her left breast since it now had a piece missing. This was the ONLY thing Mom ever expressed any dislike for: the prosthesis is a heavy piece of material with a bag type substance in her new prosthetic bra.

Mom and Dad supported the Juravinski Centre because they had been good to Mom during her treatment. They would support the various Breast Cancer events and they knew what the Cancer Centre needed.

My family had been very active in our local Breast Cancer initiatives and events since 1977. I had approached a local business owner to allow my company to partner with her in order to heighten our corporate profile in the community with women's issues, and more specifically Breast

Cancer. My young children decorated and gave out treat bags and always enjoyed the fashion show and other fundraising activities at these events. My husband Bob and our families always attended and took part by volunteering or donating prizes and gifts. It was a family affair!

Reoccurrence

Fast forward, 10 years later to NOW, and it really has become a BIGGER FAMILY AFFAIR with no time to wait to complete this project. Two months ago, Mom seemed more confused as a result of her dementia. She also appeared to have a persistent cough again and she seemed to be in some discomfort.

Since mom seemed weak, tired and more soft spoken than usual, I suggested to my Dad that we consider taking her to the hospital. What we thought was pneumonia was diagnosed at the Hamilton General as a reoccurrence of her breast cancer. The cancer had spread to her lungs. We were not at all prepared for this and neither was Mom or Dad. Her lung was so full of fluid that doctors had to drain the blood from her lungs. Next, they wanted her to follow up with an oncologist and an internist; they suggested putting a drain in her back and also explained the palliative care. WOW............really???? We were told Mom may have weeks, maybe months, and that there is little that could be done. Palliative care would keep her comfortable and out of pain. After her initial treatment years ago I thought she would remain cancer-free.

Today is August 12, 2015, her eighty-third birthday, and we have had a great day with gifts, flowers, family, children and grandchildren, treats, lunch and lots of smiles and storytelling. It was a very special day and it went the way I hoped it would. I also wondered whether this would be her last birthday. BUT something was missing: the book that I had promised to write once I retired. I have now been retired for three months, and decided to put all my effort into completing the book and sharing my story, my journey.

CHAPTER 1

THE NEED FOR THIS BOOK

"Life throws us challenges and every
challenge comes with rainbows and lights to conquer it."

When I was diagnosed the morning of my 49th birthday, February 23rd, 2009, I wanted to get as much information and resources immediately. I had so many questions that I needed answers to. What type of cancer is it? How is it treated? How sick will I become? Will I die? How will my family and others react? How will I cope? How will I look? Do I need to quit work? Is it alright to cry and be so afraid? These were some of the many questions I had and, really, I just wanted to fast forward a year and see how I survived.

On Day 2 of my diagnosis I went to Chapters in-between my medical appointments to purchase a book. I wanted to find the perfect book titled, "Everything you need to know about Breast Cancer". There was no such book. I glanced through a few and quickly read the front and back and some notes in the middle. I found books about women's cancers, holistic prevention, metastatic breast cancer, Suzanne Somers Tell-All, surgeries, mental health and cancer. I only felt depressed with all the "doom and gloom" content of these books. I wanted a book like Fran Drescher's, "Defeating Cancer with Hard Work and Humor". She wrote real and raw, but funny! I heard about this years later when she appeared on a talk show. She was the actress who appeared on the NANNY sitcom. She also refers to it as Cancer Schmancer as she embraces it with such courage, laughter and control. She stressed the need to be educated, to be a good partner with your medical team, take control of the situation and be prepared for hard work - and have fun at the same time!

Fran and I both believe and know that some of the "BEST GIFTS COME IN THE UGLIEST PACKAGES"! This is so true as I discovered so much about myself and others as a result of my cancer and the resulting struggles. I have become a stronger, simpler and more generous person. I have been empowered and more comfortable in my own skin and in my own daily choices.

I am so much more passionate and determined to educate and assist other women as they need to be aware of ALL the resources and supports; unfortunately, there are so many gaps in our medical system and within the hospitals and medical profession. My frustration has enabled me to turn all that pain and passiveness I suffered into power and empowering others.

My daughter, daughter-in-law and their daughters will have all they need in the future to fight this nasty cancer and be stronger and healthier for it. We have to enable and empower them as mothers and educators.

I recently read Jill's Journey, another book released in 2015. This is the book I needed that day in 2009 in the Chapters book store. It is simple but it deals with some of the real issues we need to know. I hope my book provides the comfort and courage that Jill's book did for so many readers. I share resources similar to her but go beyond her story with some more intimate details; this is what women are asking for and need. The hospital library and cancer clinics have the best books. They are free too as some women and families do not have the financial resources. This disease gets costly! Another issue I have with the system is the need for free resources, accessories and services for women as they fight this battle.

There are some very DARK times throughout this journey but they must happen in order to get to the lighter, happier days. We know that, but it is hard to understand when having a dark day with no end or light in sight! The title Approaching Sunrise indicates a journey to, and arrival at, the sun and a path to the better, warmer side.

"The dance between darkness and light will always remain."
C. JoyBell C.

CHAPTER 2

MY JOURNEY BEGINS

Feb 14th, 2009 - MY (not so) FUNNY VALENTINE

This has to be the most eventful Valentine's Day ever! I had felt a lump in my right breast and it hurt. It was the size of a big marble, or an alley as we called them when I was young. It moved and it was sensitive when I touched it. As I would roll in bed, it would move such that it bothered me and I could not sleep. If you can't identify with a marble, I would compare it to a large grape - but hard! I had a mammogram a few months ago so I hadn't been worried as I always keep my planned mammograms and pap smears, etc. I had a physical with my GP only a few weeks ago and she always does a breast examination so I had no reason to suspect any issues. I asked my Dr. at this time "how would you know a lump if you felt it?"

After nursing 3 children and having what I consider lumpy breasts, I can't feel what a normal lump is and what is significant to worry about. She said she would know the difference and I trusted her with that; I left my physical exam with no worries.

As this lump appeared to get bigger and really hurt, I started googling breast lumps; I called a few friends who reassured me it was nothing. I called a nurse friend and she said if it hurts, that is usually a good thing. She said not to worry but see my Dr. ASAP! I asked my husband Bob to feel it and take me seriously (as he usually doesn't get an invite to feel my breasts); he couldn't feel any big lump (as he always feels lumps) and couldn't resist copping a feel!

As much as I tried to enjoy the Valentine's and look forward to a lovely dinner out, I just couldn't relax and I was preoccupied with this lump and the thought of cancer. As it grew and became sorer I became more anxious.

It was the Family Day holiday weekend (Feb. 16th) so I was not able to get into the doctor's office (and it made no sense to go to a clinic or emergency as I needed to see Dr. Deb; she knew my breasts and knows me and my family well). I trusted her and wanted her to deal with this. I called my best friend Lois in Florida and she reassured me it would be nothing and not to panic until I see the Dr., but she understood my worry and was sensitive to what I was feeling.

Our Valentine's weekend only became more stressful as I worried about my lump.

Bob had planned dinner out at Spencer's at the Waterfront but I couldn't enjoy it. He held my hand at dinner (which he never does) and he tried to reassure me that all would be okay, but even so I got weepy.

February the 16th was Family Day, the new provincial holiday (in Ontario) for families to enjoy one another; everything was closed, including the doctor's office.

I called my doctor's office on the holiday Monday and left a crazy message for Janice, who oversees the office, and stressed the need to get me in on Tuesday! Sunday and Monday were long days. I told most of the people around me about my lump because I needed more reassurance I think, or perhaps I needed to prepare them for what might happen.

Janice called me back early on Tuesday the 17th and got me in at the first available appointment. She knew I was not going to wait. Dr. Deb agreed that there was something there because she couldn't recall feeling this a few weeks ago. She felt it needed immediate attention and referred me for a mammogram downstairs at her medical office (the same day!), and I also had to go for an ultrasound the following day. She had to have known it could be something as she got me in quick. For those of you who believe these situations don't happen and you always have to wait, that is not always the case. I have learned there is always an appointment or a way to be seen. You have to be aggressive and advocate for yourself, or for others in your family. Some of it may have been luck, but Dr. Deb knew me well enough and I trusted she would not make me wait.

I had the new mammogram and ultrasound completed on Wednesday the 18^{th,} but was waiting for a technician or radiologist to read them. How long does this take? I sought out anybody I could find to speak with to share something hopeful and positive that week. We were all downplaying it and suggesting it was nothing, but there was a look in the ultrasound technician's face that made me believe she knew something; I reacted in a way that she knew I knew. We women can pick that stuff up from other women.

Again, it was the weekend and some physicians and medical professionals were away and not working. I had to wait over another miserable weekend again, feeling my lump continue to grow bigger and more awkward when it moves. I wondered if Dr. Deb may call me over the weekend at home if she hears anything.

February 23rd, 2009 - is not just any day, it's my 49th birthday! One of my first calls of the day was from Dr. Deb, who realizes the birth date on my file; she is sick to tell me the news on the morning of my birthday. I knew it was coming: "Joanne, I am so sorry to tell you, especially today, that it looks like cancer. I am sorry." I start to swallow weird and cry, but want to know what is happening today. She explains I can pick up my disc at the facility where I had my mammogram done, and take the report to Dr. Kancherla, the Breast Cancer surgeon she recommended. It was all happening quickly (and the way I like things to go) and I will not wait because the anxiety would kill me.

I can't see Dr. Kancherla fast enough. Dr. Deb tells me the appointment will be tomorrow on Feb. 24th. I am fairly NUMB these days, and just waiting for more words, the explanations of those words and then what happens with this diagnosis. Someone (Bev) had already purchased me a Breast Cancer Journal to keep notes and appointments; I am grateful for this because I write everything down and I prefer this method rather than having everything on my computers or Blackberry. I am a writer and a visual girl. This journal has come in so handy and I have referred to it often throughout my treatment and the writing of this book. Even after treatment, follow up, (and recently because I am doing genetic testing) I needed the dates and notes in this journal.

February 24th, 2009 - My first entries in the Breast Cancer Journal were from my friends Lois and Barb.

> *"You are a very special person and I am with you all the time in my heart! Love You."* – **Lois**

"Joanne, you are so loved by all that know you. You have always been there for all of us—well It's our turn now! Please know that no matter what we need, that John and I are here for you day and night. I love you and together with our prayers and your strength you will be back to your old self real soon. We love you!" - **Barbie (special work colleague and friend) and John**.

February 25th, 2009

"We launch our battle today. We've always been strong individually, but now together with your family and many great friends, we'll get you healthy again. I love you! You are my guardian angel...but I'll wear the wings for now." - **Jeanne**

February 25th, 2009 - I saw Dr. Kancherla at 2 pm today. I worked in the morning and I also stayed late the evening as I needed to stay busy and distracted. I called Bob immediately at work after Dr. Deb called and we cried and sobbed and said we would see one another at home tonight. He told me he loved me!

Dr. Kancherla is lovely. I can tell she has seen my file which I had also read it since I picked it up for her. Of course I am going to open the file, as anyone would. I saw words like "MALIGNANT" and "GRADE III INVASIVE DUCTAL CARCINOMA". What do these words mean? All I knew was that I had breast cancer! I was somewhere between NUMB and overwhelmed and extremely afraid.

My parents wanted to come with me and I was comforted by that. Bob would have come but we did not need everyone there. We sat anxiously in Dr. K's waiting room looking at the literature and pamphlets on breast cancer and related issues. The receptionist, whom I recognize from our past somewhere, is very pleasant and friendly. I think we may know one another from our kids' past elementary school.

I get in pretty quickly and my Mom came in with me. My Dad wanted my Mom with me. I just wanted this to be explained, and decisions to be made, so that I could get rid of this mass. Dr. K reviewed why I was there, and explained briefly that we would discuss options after she looks at my lump and reviews the notes from the pathologist and radiologist. I knew what was coming and I started to feel awkward and scared. I could feel the panic as she asked me to get dressed and meet her outside in her office with my mom.

Here it comes—in her very gentle and calming way, she explains it is the most common form of cancer and is a 6cm grade 3 infiltrating ductal carcinoma and fairly aggressive. ALL I HEAR IS CANCER! She continues to explain it very calmly and slowly and about what she feels should happen. I still hear cancer! She asks if I want a second opinion. My mom is in the room and says nothing. I think she is shocked and does not know what to say. What do you say when your daughter's life is turned upside down? Is there a right response? My Mom isn't one to react and she has been through this and has had good results so I can imagine she feels I may too.

Dr. K. was thorough and felt a mastectomy was what I needed (not a lumpectomy) given the size and grade, the technician's report she had read and the mammogram she had seen. She suggests a RIGHT RADICAL MODIFIED MASTECTOMY! (Whatever all that means.) I go along with it and ask, when? She says she must look at her surgery schedule.

My mom is still quiet and showing little emotion and I anticipate falling apart when I see my Dad in the waiting room as he is more emotional. I questioned why we wouldn't remove both breasts and Dr. K. explained that there was no need, and that the other breast would help identify if cancer returned. Again, I am only hearing cancer and could not even think about a reoccurrence of cancer sometime in the future. One thing at a time.

I did get weepier when I saw my Dad, Dr. Kancherla says she may have an opening on Friday if we can get all the necessary tests done. I am thrilled as I want it done now! She says, so matter-of-factly, "if you can get the chest x-ray, bone scan and biopsy done this week, I can do surgery at 9 am this Friday." Are you kidding me? I will make sure everything is done; I am on a mission to get all these appointments organized , and fortunately I have the help of the medical secretary, whom I know as a mom from the kids' high school.

The secretary gives me a booklet and a paper with a list of all my appointment times and I am ready to go home and get ready for this. My home is a 10 minute drive from the doctor's office and we say little in the car. I want to just get home and prepare for the week and surgery and GET THIS PARTY STARTED!

We comforted one another and focused on the details, still a little weepy, and I made a pot of tea. We hadn't started to pour from the teapot, when I get a call from Dr. K's office. She has set up ALL my appointments for the week and, it all goes well, surgery is planned for *Friday, March 6th* at *9:45 am*.

February 26th - today is a noon chest x-ray, and is my pre-op at the hospital. **Friday, February 27th** is a bone scan and needle biopsy (at hospital performed by Dr. K; it is a needle inserted in the breast lump to get a sample of breast tissue). Simple! Everything going just as planned, just as I like it.

The week of February 24th was most significant, and it couldn't have been planned any better or gone any more smoothly. I must encourage those of you reading this, or who know of others experiencing this, to do the same things I did. Advocate for yourself. Insist that others advocate or be aggressive for you and demand that your tests and procedures be done as soon as possible.

Doing these things will help you get the most accurate and quickest diagnosis, as well as any second opinions that you may want or need. My doctors knew me well, and knew I could not and would not wait long as the anxiety and worry would be too much for me! We wanted to deal with as little stress as we could during this most stressful time. I was so fortunate to have the surgery a week after my diagnosis.

As I mentioned earlier, you MUST have the x-ray, bone scan, ultrasound and needle biopsy to ensure the most accurate diagnosis (the diagnosis will determine the surgery and your treatment plan). The mastectomy and pathology report a few weeks after the surgery will also provide more information about the type of cancer you are dealing with and the post-operative plan; whether it will be chemo, radiation or both. Some cancers will require chemo before your mastectomy or lumpectomy, and that will be explained to you at the time you and your surgeon meet.

The technicians were all very sensitive and aware of why we were having the tests we were having. They cannot give any opinions, but sometimes their expressions communicated things. I tried to get them to share what the tests were showing but they always keep the results to themselves.

Of all of the pre-operative procedures I had, the needle biopsy was the most frightening and uncomfortable. Dr. Kancherla spoke to me the whole time because I was awake and just frozen, but I felt a pinch of something that hurt. I believe this is one of the most important procedures as the needle is inserted into the lump to remove a small amount of the affected breast tissue. I felt okay after a local anesthetic and left the hospital with Bob soon after this quick procedure.

The week of March 1ˢᵗ is a fog but I went to work and tried to keep everything normal and on schedule. Bob was busy with high school basketball championships, and I recall attending a playoff game at Sheridan College after my bone scan and pre-op. Jamie, Zack's (my middle child) girlfriend, came to greet me in the bleachers and told me that the news has spread and "EVERYONE KNOWS!" The voice message mailbox is full and she has been responding to calls and memos from friends and family.

Jamie says it is crazy and she has started a CARE SITE so people can communicate with me online and I can receive people's wishes and notes of support. I am no "techy", and I don't really understand this and I think it is unnecessary. I don't think much more about it and try to keep interested in the game, but lots of people interrupt me to give me a hug and offer their support. Weird!

Here is the first Journal entry that Jamie started:

JOANNE'S BREAST CANCER BATTLE. (February 26ᵗʰ) www.free-webs.com/jstaceyfightforthecure/apps/blog/show/527658-thankyou-everyone-#comments (for anyone wishing to do one for themselves or a friend.)

Joanne's Story

"On February 23ʳᵈ, it was Joanne's 49ᵗʰ birthday! ……. We will keep you updated as best as we can, along with some postings by Joanne herself. Thank you for being interested in the well-being of our amazing Joanne!"

Feb. 27ᵗʰ -11:16 am - I don't recall writing but I may have dictated this to Jamie.

"It is times like these I treasure and look forward to. I am blessed to have the number of wonderful people in my life that I do! I am overwhelmed with all the wishes, emails, cards and other ways people are reaching out to me and I am surrounded with so much love, warmth and support. This is powerful and I realize how special you all are to myself and my family."
Thanks again. Love Joanne

My work week was more part-time hours as I had all these appoint-ments to attend. The staff at work were so amazing and supportive, and I knew I would be okay because I had them to lean on. I have been at my position as an executive assistant to the most wonderful boss, Jon, for 18 years, and he was so good to me during this time! I worked enough to tie up some loose ends because I was in the middle of planning a conference for mid-June.

Jack Lengyel was my keynote speaker for my event in June 2009; he is the man who was behind the story and movie WE ARE MARSHALL, (played by Matthew McConaughey). He was hired as the new football coach at the school in Huntington, West Virginia after a plane crash took the life of a college football team, as well as 40 of its community members, university staff and family members. This is still considered the greatest air tragedy in the history of athletics.

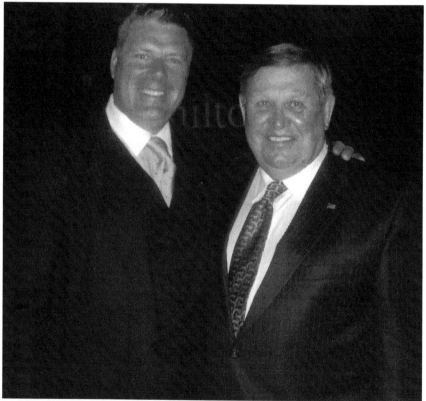

Jon Jurus (left) and Jack Lengyel, two very special men so much alike! This pic-ture is from a Sports Hamilton Event in June 2009.

Jack was hired as the new coach to recruit a new team and rebuild the football program and community. Jack gained world recognition as the "HEALER", and he dealt with the people and community who were hurting the hardest. He is known for his fight, perseverance and compassion. His motivational quotes and speeches are shared by many; he is known for his famous speech about "fighting with heart" and how it is one's heart that keeps them going and will not let them be defeated.

I couldn't have met this man at a better point; now I know things happen for a reason because he came into my life at this time! He wrote me a lovely letter and gave me a signed piece of artwork that I will cherish. One other saying of his that we can all learn from is, "Don't let difficult losses stop you before the end of your story."

He suggests pushing through whatever your crisis or loss is and uniting your team together. Pull everything that you have together to move forward. This is so true of my family and friends and my medical team. Know and trust your team!

Jack is one of the most inspirational and successful motivational speakers in the United States and I was so fortunate to have dealt with him personally. He resides in Arizona and we had been in contact with one another by phone and email confirming details of his trip and speaking engagement. I wrote him this week to let him know I would be away for a week or two.

March 3rd, 2009 at 11:29 am - Jack Lengyel wrote back,

> *"Joanne, been on the road, reading my emails backwards. Sorry to hear about your operation but would like to remind you my mother had breast cancer years ago and lived till she was 96. They are doing wonderful things today so I want you to know our prayers are with you and your family and I look forward to seeing you in June."*

Deb M., whom I knew from when some of our children attended school together, called me and asked me for lunch. She lost her son Kyle to cancer previously but Deb is so strong and her family has been such an inspiration for so many reasons. They are great community people and Hayley, Deb's daughter, is a friend to my children. Marley's Mom, Anne, came too and we went to Canyon Creek for lunch. We chose this restaurant because we all had a connection to it, and one of our friends was a manager there who wanted to see us.

After a terrific lunch and lots of catching up, we had to head home because we all had evening plans. I had my belated pre-surgery party, Anne had a contractor to meet and Deb had a dinner engagement.

On our way home we were driving behind a small car that could not stay within the road lines and was driving recklessly. Since it was 3:30 pm we were even more concerned because it was school closing time; many children were walking home while we passed two schools and knew there was one more up ahead. Anne, the driver, agreed with Deb and me that we must get beside the car to see if the driver is okay. We were shocked to find a rough looking woman, who looks intoxicated, or unwell, or under the influence of something.

We called 911 because we all felt we had to, then proceeded to follow her past our home exits going about five minutes out of our way. The dispatcher asked us to remain on the line and continue to tell her what the woman was doing and where we were. The driver had no idea we were following her, and she seemed lost as she turned into a residential area and turned around in a driveway.

We didn't know whether to laugh or cry. We can't believe this is happening; I took the CHARLIE'S ANGELS pose and told my friends in the front that I will be one of the characters, asking who do they wish to be? We started laughing madly as we continued to follow this woman and heard the siren coming towards us. The three of us were very aware of the time and were growing more concerned because we had places to be. It had now been an hour since leaving the restaurant; we were concerned about our time because we were anticipating we may have to stick around.

While we wait for the police to pull the female driver over, we took our pose that the Angels were known for, positioning their hands as if they were guns, and I snapped a photo. I always have a camera!

As frightening as this was, it was also very entertaining and we needed a laugh. The two police officers asked us to wait, but we quickly explained we couldn't stick around because we had appointments. We watched as they apprehended this poor young woman, who was definitely under the influence of drugs, alcohol or both. One police officer asked us a few questions, but then asked if they could call us later for any additional details.

They wanted us to remain at the side of the road until this was over, but we insisted we had to go and gave the officer our names and numbers.

Anne returned us all home safely and then we all met with police officers within the next few hours. This evening was my belated birthday party, as I mentioned, so I asked the officer to come early because I was home now and the other two women would be home later.

The officer was so moved by his visit with Deb because she had explained how she had lost Kyle to cancer recently, and also that I was going into surgery tomorrow for a mastectomy. He was in disbelief that we were out celebrating our friendship and enjoying the afternoon as we did despite our present challenges. I tell this story for this reason: You have to embrace the people and opportunities in your life, and celebrate the good and the blessings, because you don't know what can or may happen. We are a strength to one another and need to be comforted by one another.

Approaching Sunrise

SURGERY

I was a wreck thinking about this day. The doctors and Bob and I met to go over the procedure. As scared as I was, I was still able to take copious notes. I was still terrified of this day.

March 5th - Pre-Surgery Birthday Dinner - We finally celebrated my birthday with a fabulous birthday dinner and cancer party on Thursday, March 5th, the evening before the surgery. We wanted my daughter Natalie to be there, which meant she had to come from Ottawa where she was attending the University of Ottawa.

The night was memorable, not only as a result of our adventure that afternoon, but, because of the evening my family hosted. My children and their partners had planned a very special evening to celebrate my birthday and to support me as I was going into surgery the next morning. They put an amazing spread of food together including my favourite, lamb. Jamie, my soon-to-be daughter-in-law, orchestrated the evening and invited her family, as well as any close friends who could attend. It was a fun night; I received birthday gifts, hospital gifts, books, videos and some much needed items for the hospital and for the recovery afterwards. There were no tears - only laughter and good wishes and thoughts. It was great to have Natalie there: I needed her to be with me.

March 5th - Night Before Surgery. Blog Entry.
It is 4:06 am and the sleeping pill just isn't doing its thing for me; it's a good time to write something and view this site (this gives me great peace and a calm I cannot explain to you). Bob and I are overwhelmed with love

Surgery   1 9 and the concern of our friends and even some acquaintances and people we have never met. The strength this site has provided us is something I wish I could explain. We have all found what we needed in the kindness and generosity of others. What this beautiful network does for all who are hurting is BRILLIANT! I have learned much in this past week, including that I can be the TAKER, which is so important since I will need it. I can't be the caregiver and the glue that holds many things together. I can, however, share in all that we receive and the goodness we feel by letting others lend a hand. This is all new to me and I can only take it a day at a time.

I don't look forward and I am really scared as I have no choices and little control; I just have to embrace and accept what life has thrown at me. I have a family and a group of friends who will be there and I know I cannot do this without them. I have found HUGE comfort at this time from all of you and your words, stories and cards, chocolate, wine, flowers, gifts, but most importantly from your love and presence in my life. You have touched us in a way I have never been touched before, I am calm now and I know how blessed I am to have had this happen. I will only grow from this, and HEAL, with so much more knowledge, strength, love. And most importantly, I will be well without cancer! I still have a lot of living to do and look forward to sharing more good times with you all. I am on the sidelines for now, but know I am with you, as I need you all with me, and feel you are all wrapped around us!

Jamie is back and I think most of you know how amazing she is and has been recently. I really count on her and know how lucky we are to have her as a part of our family. Zack has been here every day and has surprised me as to how sensitive and generous he has been with me, despite his fear and feelings of shock.

Brock is struggling but came around this weekend and was part of our BACHELOR parties (reality TV). This show distracted me a bit this week! I will need Brock (a hair stylist) later for the bad hair or no hair days!

Trying to just be there for Bob, as he has been thrown into a game he is not sure how to play or coach. He needs the extra warm and fuzzies, something9+63 Johnny Mac (colleague of Bob's) was always good at recognizing and giving.

My Mom and Dad are here and want to do all they can. However I see how tough it is for them as there is only so much they can do. No parent wants to see their baby go through something like this and they have always been the caregivers. They are here and will be with me through this despite all they have gone through. My Mom had breast cancer and recently completed her treatment at Juravinski—she has done well so I expect only the same.

My brother Michael and his family, wife Lorie, daughter Alicia and son-in-law Bryan, have a beautiful granddaughter Taylor (11 months) and now have a grandson, Alexander Michael, who was born very premature. Michael Alexander fights his own battle as he weighs just less than 2 lbs. He has many challenges, but he continues to show us what a fighter he is! We will all be okay. Alexander Michael has two of the strongest grandparents in Mike and Lorie and two parents and a big sister who are so excited for him to also recover well.

Again, we don't know why bad things happen to good people, but that's okay as we are stronger for it. Lorie and I can't wait for the party and celebration our family will have when these months are over! Alicia and Bryan are two young parents who will only be empowered and enriched by this craziness, like I have. That is how we have to look at it, and laughter will get us through this too - Lorie and I had a good giggle the other morning that did us both the world of good!

So for now I close, as I need to sleep, but I will fill you in so I hope you stay tuned as I need you all here. You are a comfort, a calm and a clarity that I need during this time. I treasure you all!

Love, Joanne

Some responses to my blog on March 5th at 5 am.
Who is up at that time?

> *Lorri, one of my curling friends writes on the site*: "*My thoughts and prayers are with you and your family. I trust you will get through this. My own mom has been a survivor of breast cancer for almost 21 years. I am so happy I saw you at the club recently. You are a very strong woman and remember to be gentle with yourself as well. Love and Blessings, Lorri.*"

> *Sharon, a mom we know from our sons playing football together at University of Guelph, March 5th, 10:37 am*: "*Thank you so much for sharing your story. In reading your notes it is truly amazing how you are already "a step ahead" in knowing some of your*

feelings and knowing that laughter can truly be the best medicine. Also knowing that you have a hard road ahead, however with tons of support from family and friends and it sounds like new friends as well, know to take one day at a time which you will learn to break down into getting through the morning, afternoon, evening and night, knowing that you will have good care through your doctor, and knowing that your own mother is now one of the "famous cancer survivors", a truly wonderful accomplishment and blessing, knowing how everyone is pulling together. Part of the definition of strong is strength in numbers. Joanne, you have that for sure. Love from our family."

Kate, a friend who we met when our kids were in preschool, 10:50 am: *"As always your strength and positive approach to life is an inspiration to us all. Again, you are amazing girlfriend. My prayers and the prayers of the ladies at Wellington Square are with you, your family and doctors to rid you of all the cancer. I love you sweetie and know that God loves you even more and is with you during this time. Big hugs, Kate."*

Lois Marotta: *"It was a fateful day in February of 2009 when I got the call from Joanne that she had breast cancer. It was news that no friend wants to receive and certainly news that no one wants to relay. I cried uncontrollably at the news and finally caught my breath long enough to call my Mom for advice. You see, I was leaving the next day to fly to Florida and my best friend just delivered devastating news. What should I do? Do I stay or do I go? So Mom told me to calm down and go to see her right away. So I did! We hugged, we cried and we talked about going forward.*

From that day forward, our lives would never be the same. Yes, it was a devastating diagnosis, but what came out of it this experience was nothing but LOVE. You will get to know Joanne from reading her book and understand that she is no wallflower. Joanne is the most positive, proactive person I have ever met. Living with cancer, she never pitied herself or ever let on she wasn't going to beat this "thing". I drew from her strength, enabling me to be strong for her. I was able to hold her hand when she was scared. I was able to support her when she got her drains out but through it all, there were also lots of laughs. Joanne had this ability to make anyone feel comfortable around her and was always so open about her cancer. That openness allowed all the LOVE in. And there was a LOT of LOVE for Joanne. In fact, there was so much support for Joanne that her daughter-in-law, Jamie, had to set up a website so that anyone could get daily updates on Joanne and leave their messages of support and LOVE. What a wonderful thing!

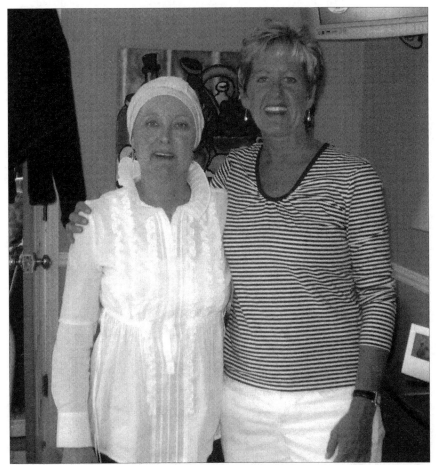

My best friend Lois and I from July 2009. Lois brought me the cap I am wearing because I started losing my hair.

Joanne has made lifelong friends whom she met through her cancer experience. So, out of something bad came something good, I'm sure Joanne would tell you that she would never wish this diagnosis on anyone, but if anyone could make lemonade out of lemons, it was Joanne. Her book will hopefully be as inspirational as she has been to me. I love you my friend! Lois Marotta."

Suzanne, a friend and colleague, 11:04 am: *"As I said to you earlier today, for everything you have been through these past two weeks, you looked amazing yesterday. I am so glad your spirits are high, keep that way always. Here are the lyrics to the song I spoke about, the only thing you need to remember is you do not have to lose (they got it wrong in the song), losing is not an option here, stay strong and know that we are here to help you climb and move that mountain."* (Miley Cyrus song) *I can almost see it. That dream I'm dreaming but there's a voice inside my head saying, you'll never reach it. Every step I'm taking, every move I make feels lost with no direction. My faith is shaking. But, I gotta keep trying, gotta keep my head held high. There's always going to be another mountain. I'm always going to want to make it move. Always going to be an uphill battle. Sometimes I'm gonna have to lose. Ain't about how fast I get there, ain't about what's waiting on the other side. It's the climb. The struggle I'm facing. The chances I'm taking, sometimes might knock me down, but, no, I'm not breaking. I may not know where. But these are the moments that I'm going to remember the most. Just got to keep on going and I, I got to be strong, just keep pushing on. There's always going to be another mountain. I'm always going to want to make it move. Always going to be an uphill battle. Sometimes I'm going to have to lose. Ain't about how fast I get there, ain't about what's waiting on the other side. It's the climb. Keep on moving, keep climbing keep on baby, it's all about the climb. Keep the faith. Love Suzanne."*

Carolyn, another colleague in another region, 1:38 pm: *"You know all of us are with you every day, in our thoughts and prayers. I have the office wearing PINK tomorrow so we can all be thinking of you. We are pulling for you, my special friend."*

ML, 7:54 pm: "Hey Sunshine… I've learned that people will forget what you said, what you did, but people will never forget how you made them feel… And Joanne, that's "why" you are so special to so many people…YOU MAKE EACH OF US FEEL SPECIAL… I am here to help you through this journey… Always, as you have been here for everyone… ML."

These are just a few of the many comments I received just that one day before surgery. The numbers are unbelievable and just continued to grow. This outpouring was overwhelming, and even awkward, as I never thought that many cared and would take the time to connect. I really didn't know that I had so many wonderful friends and acquaintances. They say that you know who your true friends are when these things happen and I am so blessed and enriched and full of so much love and support. Mind blowing!

At 9:12 pm I wrote the girls from the lunch, "To my Charlie's Angels - how much fun was that? We need those laughs and unexpected times to continue to share! FIGHTING CRIME AND BREAST CANCER AT THE SAME TIME! Fuck…….is there anything else that I can do before this craziness starts? Keep laughing as I will need it!"

Sharon (football mom), 8:51 am: "Joanne, be only as strong as you need to be today and save some of your strength for after the surgery. Let your family and friends be strong for you today and everyone will help you through this adventure."

Tracey, an old babysitter of ours and student of Bob's and good friend, 9:11 am (while being prepped for surgery): "Wow! Pretty powerful stuff! (Referring to all journal posts). You are an amazing woman Joanne, who has touched the lives of so many people. Your courage, love, strength is an inspiration…. this will truly help you along the way. Remember though that all the people around you have courage, love and strength that you can draw on too. You are well loved and a fighter. You can beat this. All my love, Trace."

March 6th - SURGERY DAY - Bob and I arrived early at Joseph Brant hospital as I just wanted to get this over with. I wanted to shower and get there and not speak with anyone or see anyone as I was so emotional and anxious. I was weepy saying goodbye to Bob; as he tells me he loves me as they take me to the Operating Room.

The nurses and admitting staff are so wonderful and compassionate as they understand what is going on inside me and in my head. They are kind and overly accommodating; one nurse recognizes me (her daughter knows Natalie) and we start chatting about our daughters. That was a nice distraction and comforting. My new friend would take extra special care of me.

Dr. K came to see me and asked if I had any questions or concerns. It is too late now I am thinking; we share a giggle and I say let's do this! I have also had the shot in my leg that has relaxed me and I am feeling good. That needle stung, so be prepared. Others said the same thing after I spoke of this surgery; no one told me before and that's probably a good thing.

As I am wheeled into the room, I can't believe how casual everything is. Nurses are speaking of their day, errands they need to do, laughing and carrying on—and I am having a breast removed! Do they know that I am having a breast removed? Are they prepared for this because I am freaking out? Their lack of interest relaxed me and then it was time to count as the anesthetist indicates he is ready to put me to sleep! This is the best part, the feeling of being HIGH after 2-3 seconds and finally, a good sleep. I haven't slept well in weeks and I know that in the past I have looked forward to being put to sleep before other surgeries. Best high ever!

I recall waking slowly and feeling heavy in my chest and wanting to just sleep. I was so dozy. I tried again to wake up as the nurses had encouraged me to do, but I was really tired and felt weird. The nurses are pleasant, the room is bright and they tell me my room is ready to be taken to. We proceed through the hospital halls (but I have no idea where we are or where we are going).

Bob was the first person I see in my room and then Natalie, Jamie, Zack and my parents. Too many people in the room but they had been waiting for me. I am in a semi-private room but the curtain is drawn so I have no idea who is there. I was in and out and groggy; I recall my friend Debbie came in as she gave me a photo of her colleagues in another office, all dressed in pink in recognition of my BC fight. How thoughtful to bring that to me as Debbie lives hours away. I didn't visit much as I was "out of it" so I am told. I find out later she has also brought me an angel sun catcher that now sits on my balcony door of my bedroom at home.

The kids tell me I am loud and swearing but I don't remember. They were concerned I was disruptive and loud for my roommate, Isabelle, as she appears to be a quieter lady. She was resting as she had surgery just before me. Her family had been with her earlier. They are all laughing at me and telling me how foul my language was but I recall nothing. Bob stays longer and everyone else leaves and he encourages me to rest and sleep. He says the surgery went well and that he has seen Dr. K; she is happy too but will get pathology results in a few weeks.

I ask Bob to pull the curtain back before he leaves so I can see my roommate and apologize to her for my behaviour and foul mouth. He does, nods at her and tells me he has met her family members, then reminds both of us to rest and that it is time for night medication. I have no idea of the time or how many hours have gone by.

Isabelle introduces me to her husband and daughter and then they all leave after Bob. She is a sweet tiny woman, soft spoken and so cute. I worry I may have offended her as she seems so quiet and I had been so loud.

Isabelle and I get acquainted and we quickly form a special bond because we have the same surgeon and had the same surgery. I joke that we are balancing the room fairly because she had her left breast removed and I had my right. Isabelle and I are pleased to be roommates and are thrilled we have one another tonight. We agree to keep the curtains open, but because I am in and out of consciousness from being tired we only speak back and forth a little. I apologize that I am not too chatty and she understood. I seemed to sleep well and had nurses come in every few hours with medication and asking me about pain. I was fairly comfortable, as was Isabelle.

The next morning we are up early, as the night shift nurses leave about 7 am and the new nurses come in. I thank those who took care of me overnight and look forward to the new shift. Breakfast comes soon after and Isabelle and I start talking about family and children, specifically our daughters, who were visiting last evening. It appears both daughters attend the University of Ottawa and they were on the same flight home to Toronto to get home to see us. What a small world! We continue to speak of our boys and their sports; Isabelle tells me her son has played against my husband's school basketball team and that she knows of Bob and his basketball program. She tells me she too is a teacher, and we continue to name more people and names of friends and acquaintances we both know. Can it get any better than this?

Dr. K comes in to the room to check on us and cannot believe how good we both look and how we are chatting away. She is pleased to see us connect as we do and reassures us we are not being discharged. I was shocked she thought we may go home because both of us have just started to walk to the bathroom with assistance, and are plugged into IVs with drains and are very uncomfortable. Isabelle tells me she would go home if Dr. K insisted, and I told her she is going nowhere. I told Isabelle to stick with me and let me do the talking and just follow my lead. I am the outspoken one, and she goes along with what I suggest and seemed relieved - as did her family!

Visitors started to come in, and we both needed assistance to wash and dress. We both wanted to get into some real pyjamas because we were still wearing the dirty hospital gowns from our surgery. We engaged in conversation with all our guests together and it was good fun and quite social. A few times I asked her if she preferred privacy and she said "NO WAY!" We really enjoyed one another and each other's friends and family. We told everyone about our daughters studying at the same school and repeated all the people we both knew in Halton, Ontario. We were having too much fun to leave and we both wanted the extra day.

I strategized as to how we could stay until Sunday, and recounted the story of why we could not go home a few times so she understood. She thought I was a character so she told me that over and over again, and was pleased I was more aggressive as she wouldn't have been that assertive.

We helped one another answer one another's phone. This was because we both had phones on the side tables on the same side our breast was removed so we couldn't answer the calls. We shared magazines and our breast cancer story. We are now sisters for life!

As the nurses, homecare workers and therapists prepped us for discharge, I remained focused on all the reasons we were in no shape to return home. The discharge planner and CCAC (Community Care Access) had not been in to see us, and we were both in rough shape and heavily medicated. I exaggerated it all as part of my strategy, but Dr. K agreed and said we could stay for one more day; they didn't need the beds and we could use another day in hospital.

I have known of many women who were forced to leave too early after one night's stay. Do not leave until you feel ready and have seen the discharge planner, CCAC, and know of your plan returning home. You will have a community nurse visit you, and will need pain prescriptions and a schedule of when bandages and the drains will be removed.

March 7th - Hospital Stay—Day 2 - I referred to this as "getting the party started" and the more I think of my stay, it did seem like a little party. It was in no way a PITY PARTY as I never really felt pity. I went through the anger, fear, anxiety, and maybe a "Why me?" but never felt sorry for myself. Isabelle was much the same and seemed to have a great attitude. We are both positive people and love life and have embraced this as part of our journey. I refer to it as a detour in my road I am travelling with a few bumps and construction along the way!

Isabelle and I felt much the same physically because we were both bandaged up and felt a little tightness and discomfort in the chest area. We both had sets of drains and tubing outside of our gowns, and we had to find ways to organize them and hide them because we didn't want our visitors to see them full of blood and liquid.

The drains collect the extra fluid that accumulates, and they are inserted through a tiny incision under the skin in the area of the breast that was removed. The number of drains can vary depending on the surgery, but we both had two. They measure what is held in the drains because they cannot be removed until there is very little or nothing left inside. The nurse you see once you return home will monitor this and take them out when you are ready. Sometimes drains are kept in longer, and the surgeon will take the drain or drains out at a follow up appointment.

This is where pyjamas with pockets came in handy; I placed the drains in a pocket. Some patients have pinned a drain to their clothing too. A pillow was helpful to place under the arm of the side of the breast removed because it offered support and comfort.

Because I had lymph nodes removed, I felt some numbness on my right arm, shoulder and the side of my chest. I just knew that whole right side felt weird and I couldn't move it or feel it. Dr. K had told me I would feel like this and would have to exercise and receive some therapy and/or attend some classes. The nurses and CCAC discharge lady also mentioned stretching and shower exercises. Isabelle and I reviewed some of the things we were told, but we really wouldn't do anything until we got home and learned more. Then we would respond as we discovered just how we felt, what we were able to do, and when we could see what the results were of these surgeries we had both had.

Below is a picture of a breast after a mastectomy. As I mentioned earlier, I wish there was a book when I was confronting this that showed me the realities of the situation.

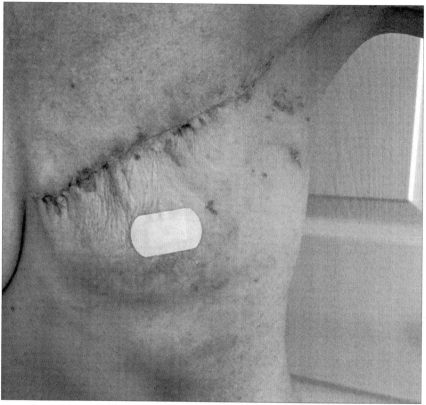

Here is a picture of a breast two weeks after a mastectomy.

She was afraid of what may become of all this, more noticeably than anyone else. I told her I couldn't worry about her and she reminded me again that it wasn't just about me. She repeated that she was afraid of what may come of all this and I tried to reassure her and others that it will be okay; I know it affects all of us. Now they have lovely drain camisoles and bras that have an insert for the drains. My friend Julie has a store in Hamilton, Ontario, and she was one of the first I was aware of who carried these camisoles. I would get to know Julie well over the next few months because she fit my prosthesis. My friend Barb, at Mount Royal Plaza in Burlington, and Julie, on Ottawa Street in Hamilton, provide them to surgeons. How very generous of them! Also, I would be going to Florida in the spring so I would need a special bathing suit, and Julie could help me with this. I will explain more about this later when it fits in sequence with the rest of my story.

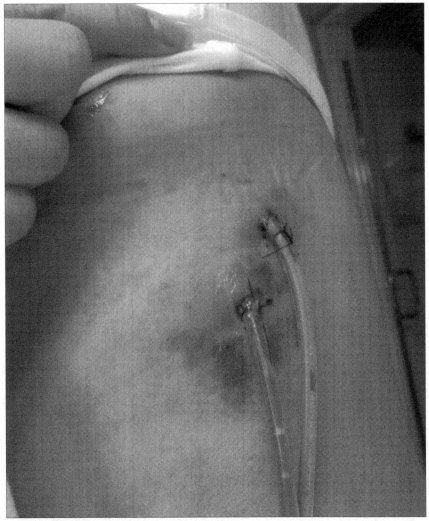

This is a picture of me post-op with two drains.

The room is starting to fill with more visitors, more flowers, more gifts and more fun. Isabelle and I are both recovering well and enjoying our time together, despite the journey ahead for us. It was easier to think and be in the moment, rather than the unknown future!

Speaking of the future, neither one of us was entertaining reconstruction anytime soon - we would think about that after getting through this experience first. Dr. K and some friends had encouraged reconstruction, but I could only consider one surgery at a time. This was because I was so overwhelmed and panicked just with the cancer surprise and diagnosis that there is no way I could have thought about reconstruction and all that is involved with that. I wasn't given the option of having both surgeries at the same time - I wanted the cancer surgery right away, and an appointment with a plastic surgeon would have taken months, if not longer. The waiting list for my plastic surgeon now at the Hamilton General is 2-3 years.

This is where my friend Jeanne enters this story. She wanted me to consider undergoing reconstruction because she said, "You have to feel good about the new year and so far you do not."

This is where we as the patient need to recognize the impact our cancer has on others! Jeanne was very emotional and joked a few days after the diagnosis that, "This isn't just happening to you." Jeanne was a mess and found it really hard to talk to me about my cancer.

Similar to me, Jeanne likes to be in control and doesn't deal well with chaos and a crisis she has no control over. She was afraid of what may become of all this, more noticeably than anyone else. I told her I couldn't worry about her and she reminded me again that this just wasn't about me. She cried: I don't see her like this often. She and I have handled crisis well in the past. Most recently she had a seizure in a park close to my home; I just happened to be attending a meeting by the park and saw her son waving me down while waiting for an ambulance. I seem to always be around when she needs me, and we have a silly belief that I am here to serve as her guardian angel or fairy godmother or someone who always is there for her. Now she has to be there for me, and as she said in one of my first journal postings, "She will wear the wings now" to take care of me.

Lois had to return to Florida but will return soon because she has other engagements back here in Mississauga. A few friends came to visit, but not too many; I prefer to see them when I return home tomorrow. I don't think Dr. K will give us another day. We have been in for two overnights and a third day. Some people have told me their friends were out the next day with drains and much discomfort - ridiculous! Ladies, speak up!

You need to stay until you are comfortable, and know what happens when you get home. If the CCAC homecare supervisor hadn't come to see us and explained our home care and what to expect when we are discharged, I wouldn't have left. Isabelle and I only had our IVs taken out that morning before we left, and hadn't met with CCAC until just before we were discharged. The nurses on the floor had to give us our post-surgery literature and medication requisitions, and other things. Isabelle was getting organized and ready before me, so I knew we were really going today; we would have to leave this safe and fun room where we were taken care of, accommodated, had our questions answered and our doctors and safety net were at pretty close reach. We now had to go our own ways and discover what this NEW NORMAL and new look was all about.

We have one another for support yet we have no real direction, or know what we are doing once we get home. We know we should exercise, perhaps see a therapist, or attend a program (as lymphedema may set in). We can contact Juravinski or our wellness centres for support and follow up, see our new oncologist for the next rounds of treatment, and maybe consider reconstruction or a naturopath or massage - so much to consider!

Natalie is staying home this semester: she has chosen to stay with me and not return to her second term at U of Ottawa. Natalie is going to be my own private nurse. Did I want her to give up her program for the semester? No, but i was thrilled she did. I was hard on her at times, and I didn't realize it until she told me. I forgot how this was affecting her, how worried she was about me and what the future may hold.

Natalie wanted me to fight and constantly reminded me of that. Our kids worry and when they see us weak and ill, they worry we may not heal or that we will give up. They have no control over our illness and can only encourage and support our healing and treatment.

All my children felt helpless and could only comfort me with their time, love and taking care of me. They oversaw the household chores and did everything I asked, despite how demanding or miserable I may have been. My parents and Bob behaved the same and did anything for me, as did my friends.

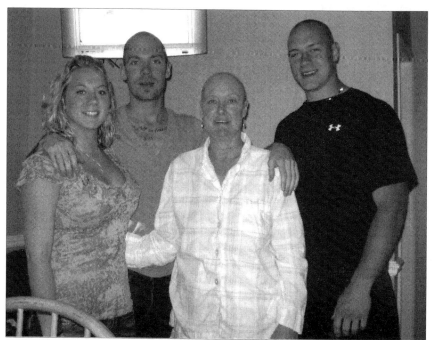
Me with my amazing kids, Natalie, Brock and Zackary.

As I have said earlier, accepting the help of others was the most difficult thing. To feel weak and needing to be dependent on others is not something I do well.

I got better at it as my treatment and illness progressed because I had no choice.

Having family and friends dress you, feed you, help you bathe and dress is tough - this was a huge shift for me, but it prepared me for more to come (you will understand as you read on).

March 9th - I'm Back! First blog entry since surgery! This is Joanne, at Natalie's laptop........Sunday night – good to be back home! As you heard from my site, I was able to stay another night as I wasn't well and we weren't ready to leave. How they allow a woman to go home after a day, I have no idea. I was sore, in pain, dizzy, emotional and uncomfortable with these new drains, unsure of the meds, anxious and still so overwhelmed.......

I have made a very special friend, Isabelle, my roomy who also had a mastectomy. What a comfort having someone else go through the same thing and same feelings. We shared laughs and so many neat things – what a small world! Our daughters both attend the University of Ottawa and took flights 40 minutes apart to come see their mothers! Isabelle's son played basketball at the Halton finals last week and we were there too since Bob's team played after their game. So many other little things we had in common that really don't matter.....but they were comforting.

What matters is that our surgery is over and it went well for both of us and we are returning home. Dr. K feels good about both of us—she feels she got all my cancer and took lymph nodes that needed to go too. I will see her next week to have drains removed and she can see the incision and how it is mending. We will discuss treatment, chemotherapy for sure and maybe radiation.

The community nurse will come tomorrow—I will need her every day.

My family has been here all week and Lois arrives tomorrow from Florida, so I am well taken care of.

To all of you who have been there for us, I can't say enough to THANK YOU for the generosity, kindness, love and support you have shown. It got us through one of the roughest times and I know we have rougher days ahead.

What you all did is so special and we are blessed to have you in our lives. We have found a calm and relief from this site and feel empowered as did many others. You have embraced us when we needed your caring, your prayers, your understanding, your patience and your love. I am tired and will write more later. Good night, Joanne.

A few significant notes from friends March 10th-11th,

> **ML writes** - *"Hey sunshine....I've learned that people will forget what you said, forget what you did, but will never forget how you made them feel...And Joanne that's why you are so special to so many people...You may each of us feel special. If I can help in any way through this journey know I am here...Always...as you have been there for everyone......ML"*

> **Laura P.** – *"Hi Joanne! It has been a long time since we chatted. I am so happy to hear that everything went well. I have been think-ing of you all weekend. It was a miracle to have someone in your room that is going through the same thing. It must have made your stay more comfortable. You are an amazing woman! Good luck*

with the treatments and healing. I am wishing you a fast recovery. Take care my friend."

Amazingly, it turned out that Laura would be diagnosed with breast cancer 5 years later - we reconnected through this site and her cancer. This site helped her and I was able to be there for her 5 years later!

Vivian writes- "*I am not surprised that you found someone in your room who shared so much with you. For as long as I known you, you have drawn people to you. You are the organizer, planner and coordinator. I know you did not schedule this into your life. I know your positive attitude and generous spirit will help you get through this. Let others coordinate and tie up the loose ends while you rest and get your strength back. No one and NOTHING can keep a spirit of yours down for long."*

March 10th & 11th - were resting days and visitors. My family rearranged the fridge and freezer as a result of all the foods being delivered. Nat and Jamie were preparing platters of treats and fruits as we received so many fabulous Edible Arrangements. The most emotional visit was from Deb and Hayley McMillan, Kyle's family. They had made cupcakes to bring over. They also gave me a clipping of the saying Kyle had included in his journal as he fought cancer, "QUIET ALL DOUBTS".

For them to share this with me was precious and personal, especially since his passing is still so fresh and they are still healing. Those words of Kyle's were beautiful and inspiring. The clipping sits in a frame in my living room ever since they gave it to me, and I have reminded many others of it.

This blew me away and demonstrates the courage and strength Kyle possessed during his battle, and how he demonstrated a great will and passion for life.

This is so similar to what the wise Jack Lengyel had said about fight, perseverance and compassion and "fighting with heart". Jack said, "Don't let difficult losses stop you before the end of your story". Young Kyle had a beautiful story and told it until the end and we are a part of his story that remains today. We have learned so much from Kyle and his family and the effect they have had on me is significant.

CHAPTER 4

THE UNVEILING

FRIDAY the 13ᵗʰ - THE UNVEILING - The past days were busy but enjoyable, seeing so many people. Marg, my nurse, was coming to take the bandages off my chest and the drains out. I had no idea what to expect and how this would affect me.

Looking back, this was, and will be for many, one of the most emotional days since diagnosis. My journal entry does not capture the enormity of this day but I will try.

I knew my terrific nurse was coming by early to remove dressings and look at the drains and incisions. To be prepared I showered and dressed in one of my many lovely lounging outfits. I became so anxious to see this; my stress increased as Marg unpacked her tools, placed her gloves on and got closer. My body was tight and I could not relax. Most days we were downstairs in the den where I was the most comfortable. Bob always prepared a fire, and it was cozy. It was out of the way of the louder main floor, and far less busy and quieter. Today we needed this privacy and calm, knowing this undressing would be difficult - seeing my chest with no breast for the first time with scars and drains, etc.

Natalie asked if she was needed and whether she should be present, and I said yes. Marg crouched down closer and in front of me, and very gently started taking bandages off. I slowly removed the additional buttons on my pajama top as I thought it might need to be fully removed. As Marg so very gently removed the gauze, I felt the tears run down my cheek. I was staring at Natalie or the wall, just anywhere but down at my breasts. As Marg peeled the last dressing off, and as the tears flowed more and I was sad, we heard movement upstairs. It was LOIS who incredibly appeared in front of me and took my hand. We could not have planned that any better! Why do these amazing things continue to happen the timing of such significant events and people? I have to believe someone is watching – my angels!

I am crying, Nat is crying, Lois is crying, and in her most calm and reassuring voice, Lois says, "It really looks good." Marg agrees. Good, I think, but how can that be? I have lost a breast. I am deformed and a big piece of me is gone.

What do Lois and Nat really think as they come closer to look and comfort me? I wish I had seen a photo of what this may look like to prepare myself. I have no idea what to expect, or when to look.

As much as I had prepared myself and read books and asked questions, NEVER are you prepared for this. There are NO resources or HOW TO FEEL books when this happens. I eventually went to a mirror to see what I looked like. I cried and had one of those moments. I felt awkward and unbalanced, but I knew it was best to be without a breast full of cancer. I worried about how Natalie felt seeing me disfigured with ugly red scars and no breast. What was Lois really thinking? Remember to let others in your world tell you how they may be feeling because they have fears for you and are worried for you. They too are sad.

Not having the fear and worry of having cancer provided me with some comfort though. I was comforted with Lois and Marg there, and of course Natalie too. Marg took one drain out but the other remained because fluid was still draining.

We had some tea and spoke of my next appointment with Dr. Kancherla on March 17 (St. Patrick's Day), and I was anxious to get the pathology results. I was also keen to move onto the next part-treatment.

The appointment at Juravinski is April 3rd, 2009. Lois and I enjoyed some fruit and dessert from many of the Edible Arrangements and pastries people have sent. These times with Lois are precious; she has flown here from Florida to be with me! She helps me prepare for what lies ahead and keeps me organized, as things are overwhelming for me right now. She makes suggestions and, as I feel she is knowledgeable and very sensible, I trust her more than anyone. Lois encourages me to consider looking for a prosthetic bra and she offered to take me shopping as I cannot drive.

March 28th - Journal entry - Since this is my new journey, which may be the toughest, I thought this ANGEL Calendar (I received this from Dianne and Jeff, Investors Group colleagues from London.) may come in handy while at the Juravinski at my chemotherapy sessions.

I have always feared cancer, as most do. What I feared more was chemo. I thought NEVER ME! All these journals and stationery and various books have been so therapeutic and precious and such practical gifts. I use them and need them. The Angel calendar is so special; I was drawn to the March 15th entry I have mentioned so many times: "Wrap your wings around my heart and heal me from my pain and fear". This says it all and my family and friends are those angels.

March 17th entry on calendar reads. "*Today my mountain seems impossible to climb. But I know, with unseen helpers, I will climb upward fearlessly and courageously overcoming every roadblock in my path and eventually conquer them all, having become a stronger, better person.*" I truly believe that this illness and treatment and all I will go through and learn will empower me and open me up to so much more. I am starting to get it!

In my *I AM NOT MY BREAST CANCER* book that Lois bought me, one survivor writes, "*I would venture to add though that if you listed the benefits, since you first became ill with breast cancer, they would outweigh the negatives.*" I can say that the smaller things that did not mean much to me years ago are now magnified for me and have become more significant to me now than back then. It is unfortunate that it takes a crisis for us to understand what it is really important when it should be simpler.

April 1st- APRIL FUCKIN' FOOLS - I wish this was all a prank. I could not get to work today despite my effort. I showered and tried to dress but my body said no. Maybe I am doing too much. I feel I need to rest as much is happening and I am tired. I am anxious for this Friday, for chemo to start. I am ready and the sooner it starts the sooner it is over, so *Let's Get This Party Started*!

Despite what I said about books and reading too much, I am comforted by some of them and, most important, I have educated myself. Others agree that education and understanding what was happening and having some control was significant.

Here are a few things I wish to share that helped me through my journey:

"The anger and fear are so close and sometimes I am scared. I think all these have a healthy place in the healing but the problem is when one or the other take over."

"Things I trusted are gone. What really upsets me is the realization that nothing will ever be the same. I feel vulnerable, angry, frustrated, and exposed and I hate it." This was huge for me!

One woman wrote, *"I learned it's possible to be strong and sad at the same time! I hate that no matter what I do, I will never have my body back to what it was."* I needed to know what I was thinking was the same as them and that it is ok.

"I hate that I have become wiser through this. I hate that my children have had to see this and I really hate that I may have passed this on to my daughter...... But most of all, I hate that every time I get sick or don't feel well, my poor kids begin to worry now because cancer put that fear in their hearts and I now it will be a long time before they get past this and that breaks my heart."

"Cancer has made us understand that bad things do happen to good people. I hate that at this moment, there are women freaking out at just having heard their breast cancer diagnosis. I hate that my husband has to live the rest of his life without boobs."

Lastly, I agree with what most of these women had to say. I agree too that how we choose to deal with our fear and our cancer is uniquely ours! I fear not living my life the way I had chosen to live it. I fear these things I am experiencing may prevent me from moving forward with my good life. Fear motivates me to fight this disease. I cannot control the disease but I can control my fight and I trust my team to get me through this. I can be the best caretaker of my body to help my team and myself fight this cancer and the effects of treatment. I can control and assist in my healing and successful recovery. That empowers me.

CHAPTER 5

CHEMO BEGINS

This week has been stressful; I am anticipating chemo and am anxious, thinking only of the worse.

April 3rd - Clinic D with Dr. Tozer. My first visit with my oncologist; Bob, Mom and Dad were there too. Dr. Tozer explained very thoroughly how he would oversee my treatment for the next year.

He examined me and thought my scar and healing looked great, which made me feel good. He asked me if I had any questions and he noticed the questions in my journal; he picked up my book and answered every question. I thought this was brilliant and very kind and sensitive. He suggested someone else takes notes, but I wrote down everything he said since I didn't want to miss a thing.

We then went to the pharmacy and picked up $3400 worth of Neupogen injections that needed to be refrigerated. Be prepared for the costs of medication; contact your insurance company and come with a credit card that has room on it as the costs can be high! We had no idea of these costs or that I had to give myself injections. I needed these as my white bold cell count was low and chemo would weaken my immune system. The Neupogen is preventative and helps to fight infection.

April 7th - I worked until 3 pm and needed to keep busy at work to keep my mind off the chemo tomorrow. I stopped at the grocery store as Natalie was making a very healthy pre-chemo dinner. We all watched American Idol and I wanted to try to get a good sleep, so I took 2 sleeping pills.

April 8th - First Chemo Treatment - Natalie and I ran errands and went to the Bulk Barn to pick up trail mix and almonds and fruits. We arrived at the cancer clinic about 1 pm and checked in to the chemo suite. I was pleasantly surprised that Bob's cousin Stu showed up. He had been in chemo earlier that year and wanted to be there for me to explain ALL that was happening and to offer me his support and laughs. He recalled his first treatment and he knew very well my fears and worries; he made Natalie and me feel so much better. He was a very entertaining distraction.

Natalie and I could not believe how fast the treatment went. I felt OK and the treatment was more comfortable and less frightening than I thought it would be. I believed the IV would be more difficult and would hurt, but Michele my nurse was so gentle and very kind and sensitive to my anxiety and fear. My friend Joy, the nurse who did the orientation I attended with Barb, was in the chemo suite this day and she had asked Michele to take good care of me. That offered me some reassurance and relief. Natalie felt better that Joy was there and came by to speak with us.

Our nurse Michele explained everything about the chemotherapy very well so that we understood. Anything else we needed to know, Stu, who had just completed chemo, told us—and much more. I recall Stu telling us not to be surprised if I pee red as that was the chemo drug coming out. Nobody had told him so he made sure I knew. I appreciated that as that would have been a shock! The nurse explained ALL the side effects, but she said she was not worried about me feeling them all, if any.

Michele outlined all the complications and difficulties with chemo; she has to by law as the patient needs to be aware. Much of this was covered in the orientation and the many pamphlets I had read recently. **Sadly, not much was mentioned in books, and that is why I am writing this.** The vomiting and mouth sores were the two side effects I really was afraid of. I am lucky I have never been someone who vomits. I tend to ice myself or hyperventilate before I will make myself sick. I have never been comfortable with vomit or seeing others vomit. I have never had mouth sores or cold sores so this bothered me.

I went to the bathroom twice with my IV pole while having chemo. Stu told me I could and I felt so comfortable moving and having chemotherapy at the same time. Without his help I don't know if I would have attempted the washroom the first time. I prepared myself well for chemo and drank way too much; I was so worried I wouldn't drink enough, something as they had mentioned at the orientation.

My journal suggests I was "tingling" while having chemo and light headed. I felt good getting some fresh air while walking to the car after treatment. As long as I can remember, whether I drank too much or felt nauseous, I always felt better with an ice pack or going to a cool place. To this day, I do the same and find a cooler spot or need to be in the fresh air.

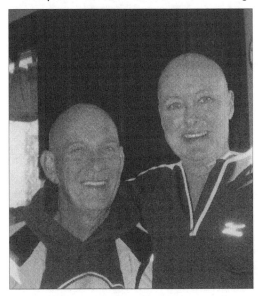

Me and my cousin Stu who was also receiving chemo at the same time. He came to visit me to raise my spirits and give me hope. A wonderful man who we lost just over a year later in 2010.

I was pleased Natalie was with me the first time. She seemed to feel better with Stu there, and didn't seem to mind being in the chemo suite seeing me receive treatment. She is the toughest of my three children when it comes to hospitals and needles.

(Journal entry)

"Tonight, I am nauseous with a headache but that is better than what I had expected it to be. I was able to eat a small dinner of salmon and salad and I kept it down—I was worried I may throw it up. I was drinking a lot of water too, as I was told to. I have rinsed with the Biotene mouthwash several times already because I am so paranoid about the mouth sores. I have brushed my teeth twice already after snacking since they suggest more thorough care of the gums with chemo. It's a good thing I have focused on my dental work the past year with fillings, a crown, cleanings, etc.

My eyes are sore and dry. We had a quiet evening, watched TV and went to bed after I took the meds and sleeping pill at 10:30 pm. I only got a good 5 hours with the sleeping pill. I was up at 5 am to go to the bathroom but went back to sleep until 7:30 am."

April 9th - Journal entries from Angel Journal - "Rougher day! Light headed, nausea, weak and little appetite. I ate some bits and pieces and still eating fairly well. Spent most of the day in bed. I didn't wish to be around people. Marg, my nurse, is coming tomorrow to do my Neupogen injection."

April 10th - **(Good Friday)** - Not so good as Nat writes on the care site. Bad day and spent half of it in bed. I got up at 11 am as Marg was coming over; Bev (a friend very active in our BC community) was dropping by too. The family was all together for dinner, and happily Nat prepared everything before she returns to Ottawa tomorrow.

Bed at 9 pm, took sleeping pills about 11 pm and slept well right through to 6 am. Weak, but not feeling as bad as yesterday. Still nauseous but managing better. Rinsing with Biotene mouthwash as I am so worried about the mouth sores. Had a bowel movement, so that was good!

April 11th - (*Day 4 after chemotherapy*) - Felt a little better—got up at 8 am and showered and I got dressed out of my pyjamas. Even felt well enough to have Natalie drive me to the bank, run errands and do groceries. I will miss her as it has been so good to have her around right now. She is back in three weeks.

Lois called from Florida to tell me she found a great site for turbans and that they specialize in mastectomy/chemo beanies and caps. I ordered some and Lois will bring them when she visits in 2 weeks. They are coming from a company in Dallas (Head Covers) so we can save the US shipping costs if they are sent to Lois. I could not find soft, attractive cotton caps locally so Lois found these for me. (You can find them locally now.)

It is 1 pm and I am relaxing now as I have had enough activity today. Marg is coming at 4 pm for my Neupogen injection. It is her day off but she is doing it to help me; I cannot do these myself like they expect you to. I am so lucky to have Marg as my CCAC nurse. (Community Care Access Community). They suggest a member of the family doing it. We could not do it and couldn't believe they were suggesting it. Bob is so uncomfortable with needles, as am I. Never did I think I would have to administer an injection to myself.

April 12th - Rough morning, feeling sick and a bad stomach. Able to have a necessary bowel movement, which is exciting these days. I don't want to be constipated, vomit or have mouth sores. Those are the 3 side effects I can't have. I got up about 7 am and made pancakes as I had a craving for syrup. I had some fruit too. I am rinsing with baking powder too to keep these mouth sores away. I got a burst of energy that I needed to get out of this "slump" as I try to take some control of this exhaustion I feel. I painted a kitchen door. That was good but I needed a rest. I had a shower about 9 am and did my hair and got dressed. I may not have hair soon so I better enjoy it while I can.

My body is aching and I could take a pain pill. Fingers a little tingly but they said this could happen. Marg called and said she would be here at 11 am. She is great and we just talk and talk. I always have coffee and a dessert ready for her. We spoke more about my mental state and how very difficult this is for me! I gave Marg some red wine (she really enjoys it); she has been so very good to me, especially coming over on her days off. She helped Bob do an injection but it didn't go well. The closest he has come to an injection is an epipen. As a teacher he knows to use one if a student has an allergic reaction but he has never had to administer one. He jammed me hard in my upper leg and it hurt. He hated it, and was so uncomfortable, but we had to try since they expect either you to do this yourself or have someone in the family do it for you. Bless him for trying, especially as he is so awkward with needles. Marg will suggest to the agency that I need her or another nurse to do the injections as we are just too uncomfortable. I would not even try!

I had some ham, yogurt and watched SAVE THE LAST DANCE. I seem to want to watch sad films or love stories lately. I called Natalie in Ottawa and she was watching it too! I just can't watch anything to do with cancer or illness so I won't be watching STEPMOM.

JoAnne Porter made our Easter turkey with dressing, gravy, dessert, and all the trimmings! What a very special friend and generous gift! I don't know what I would do without her and others like her. I had a rough morning as I am really down. I called Lois to tell her how much I missed her. Also told her I had not confirmed my order of turbans or cancer caps with the Dallas company she found for me. I had ordered them but had not received a confirmation. I am anxious to receive those caps as I need to cover this bald head and haven't found any comfortable caps yet locally. I haven't looked that hard either though since I haven't felt like going out.

[The following two pages outline my personal chemo schedule. Your oncology team provides you with the schedule outlining the medication and explaining your chemo regiment. I added these two pages because prior to receiving them I was very anxious and overwhelmed with how to organize and understand the treatment schedule. I wish I had this as part of the pre-op meeting]

AC/T DOSE DENSE Group 1 Chemotherapy

This Chemotherapy is used to treat Breast Cancer
- The treatment is given every 14 days (2 weeks).
- On Day 3 start injecting subcutaneously Neupogen once daily for 8 days from Day 3 to Day 10

Day 1	Day 2	Day 3	Day 4	Day 5	Day 6	Day 7
IV Chemo		Neupogen injection	Neupogen Injection	Neupogen Injection	Neupogen Injection	Neupogen Injection
30 minutes before chemo: Take 1 tab(1mg) of Granisetron **and** 5 tabs (20mg) of Dexamethasone	**In the morning after breakfast** Take 1 tab (1mg) Granisetron **and** 2 tablets (8mg) of Dexamethasone	**In the morning after breakfast** Take 1 tab (1mg) Granisetron **and** 2 tablets (8mg) of Dexamethasone				
'n the evening: ake 1 tab (1mg) Granisetron	**In the evening after supper** Take 1 tab (1mg) Granisetron **and** 2 tablets (8mg) of Dexamethasone	**In the evening after supper** Take 1 tab (1mg) Granisetron **and** 2 tablets (8mg) of Dexamethasone				
Day 8 Neupogen Injection	**9** Neupogen Injection	**10** Neupogen Injection	**11**	**12**	**13**	**14**

Granisetron = Kytril – for nausea – Take 1 tablet (1mg) 30 minutes before chemo treatment on Day 1 and 1 tablet every 12 hours starting the evening of chemo treatment for 5 doses

Dexamethasone – for nausea– Take 5 tablets (20mg) 30 minutes before chemo treatment on Day 1 then take 2 tablets (8mg) twice a day (in the morning and evening) starting the morning after chemo for 4 doses

Prochlorperazine = Stemetil – for persistent nausea –Take 1 tablet (10mg) every 4 – 6 hours if needed

Jatrovinski Cancer Centre
A simple Cour Ontario regional partner

Prepared by JCC Pharmacy Department   *Version date: May 2010*

AC-T DOSE DENSE GROUP 2 (Paclitaxel) Chemotherapy

This Chemotherapy is used to treat Breast Cancer

- The treatment will take approximately 4 hours to infuse.
- Two days after your chemo treatment (day 3), you will start receiving Neupogen injections (1 injection per day) for 8 days. Neupogen is used to stimulate the growth of white blood cells.
- You will need to have your Dexamethasone filled a day prior to your Paclitaxel treatment as the drug is used to prevent reactions from the treatment.

The day before chemo	Day 1 IV Chemo	2 The day after chemo	3 Neupogen	4 Neupogen	5 Neupogen	6 Neupogen	7 Neupogen
In the morning: Dexamethasone 2 tablets(8mg) **In the evening:** Dexamethasone 2 tablets(8mg)	**In the morning:** Dexamethasone 2 tablets(8mg) **In the evening:** Dexamethasone 2 tablets(8mg)	**In the morning:** Dexamethasone 2 tablets(8mg) **In the evening:** Dexamethasone 2 tablets(8mg)					
8 Neupogen	9 Neupogen	10 Neupogen	11	12	13	14	

Dexamethasone = Decadron – for nausea and allergic reactions prevention – Take 2 tablets (8mg) twice daily for 3 days starting the day before chemotherapy treatment.

Prochlorperazine = Stemetil – for nausea –Take 1 tablet (10mg) every 4 – 6 hours as needed

April 12th continued - Mom and Dad came over with cooked vegetables and Bob and I made the potatoes. I still can't believe JoAnne made 2 turkeys, one for us and one for her own family! She is so thoughtful and would do anything for me. Zack was given Raptor tickets from our friends the Simiones so he will need to leave early. Brock is dropping by and Nat is in Ottawa so this is a different kind of Easter—but everything is a little different now.

April 13th (Easter Monday)- I went to work for 3 hours today (I also did some hours last week) and this is good for me. Jon is so patient and sensitive to the treatment and the surgery and what I am able to work. When I do too much, I feel it. I have little appetite and am a little light headed at times. I get about 5 hours sleep but need more time in the morning as I ache. I can't rush and if I do I get frustrated. Bob sleeps in the spare room as I am agitated at night and disruptive and need to watch TV or get up.

Marg has done my Neupogen injections all week but has to discharge me this Friday (the 17th) as they won't allow her to continue to do them. We are so anxious about these injections! Oriol, my neighbour who is a nurse, has volunteered to do my injections; we are so relieved and so appreciative, as this was causing me huge anxiety. I had to miss our Region meeting at work since I needed the last injection of my first chemo cycle. I could not do a full day in Toronto either. I was disappointed as I always enjoy these. Also, I was being discharged from Marg, so that was something I needed to be there for. I went out to lunch with Jean, a friend on the PFLAG [Parents & Friends & Family of Lesbians & Gays] board I sit on, so that was really nice. The fresh air was great and it was about 60 degrees. I still like to think of temperature this way and not Celsius.

I felt a small sore on the inside of my lower lip and started to freak out! Was this a mouth sore they talk about? Marg thinks I am overreacting and believes it to be a coincidence and not a chemo sore. Marg thinks I am brushing, flossing and rinsing too much as I am so paranoid about these sores. The gums are so sensitive during chemotherapy so I could be rinsing too much. They warn you not to floss during chemo too!

I am also feeling more aches and spasms in the top of my legs.

Bob and I went to Pearl Street café for dinner and walked around downtown Burlington, which was really nice. We arrived home about 8 pm and I felt more tightness in the middle of my back and in my chest. It bothered me so I decided to run a bath as I needed to calm down. I scared myself so I asked Bob to sit with me and reread my pamphlets and booklets to make sure I was okay and that these aches were normal.

My body cramps got tighter while I was in the bath so we reviewed all the reading materials and reviewed the side effects of chemo and what to do. Bob is so patient; he just sat with me as I had asked. His presence was just calming, as there was nothing he could do. This is difficult for him; he is helpless and has no idea what I am feeling and how to comfort me. It is so important to remember that our spouses or partners do feel helpless and worry about us.

I know he was afraid but I tried to reassure him I would be OK and tried to be tough. I went downstairs, despite my pain, and found more booklets to read. They mentioned abdominal cramps and chest pain so I felt relieved. They mentioned that you should call the oncology department or 911. However, it was 10 pm and Bob was asleep beside me and I didn't feel we needed 911.

As I reread my many notes, it had also indicated red dots on the skin as a result of the low blood platelets. I looked all over my body and I did found dots on my upper legs. Sometimes we shouldn't read all these books; as it can make you worry unnecessarily and you start to look for all the side effects. I do have a very small mouth sore, but I agree with Marg that it may be a result of too much flossing and rinsing (I am doing it 3-4 times a day).

I called JoAnne (my turkey cook) and we had a few laughs even though it was late, and she made me feel better. She reassured me that all these aches and sores were just a result of all the new medication and the SHOCK my body is under. I just took 2 Tylenol for the discomfort and 2 sleeping pills as I need to sleep. I rinsed again before bed.

We have chosen to sell our house and the real estate agents had called: we have 2 showings tomorrow.

My injections don't start until next Friday (see chart), 2 days after chemo. Oriol will do them; we will work together to accommodate her schedule as we are so grateful she is doing them. Marg will do them if Oriol can't. This is so generous of them. I know Marg will continue to drop by as we have developed a friendship over this time. We enjoy one another and I am in her work area. We gave Marg some gifts when she discharged and she was very appreciative. She became a very special part of this new journey - she will remain a special person and she will be in touch.

I am having bowel movements so at least I am not constipated. This is a worry when taking pain meds, so take the stool softeners at the same time. I have a sore throat so I suck my Ricola lozenges and drink more tea. I am eating more bran in the mornings, as the oncology people suggest, usually with yogurt and fruit. This has become my breakfast routine and I am also drinking some prune juice and Ginger ale as the dietician recommends. Ginger ale for nausea and prune juice to poop.

My parents left for Florida and arrived safely to the house in Deerfield Beach.

April 24th - A good day, considering they say DAY 3 is usually the worst in this chemo round. I am nauseous but that is OK. Oriol came at 8 am for my injection. I had bran and fruit for breakfast since that has been working well. I spent some time on the computer searching MLS listings as we need to find a home. Good lunch of roast beef and melted cheese—my appetite is great! A friend who hadn't seen my pixie cut yet came over for a visit—she loved it. Nurse Marg called and hopes to come to visit today.

I felt well enough to start packing some moving boxes of glasses and crystal. Jamie came for a visit. I am surprised I feel this well as I should be nauseous. I have no headaches or muscle aches either. I believe keeping active, not dwelling on what should happen and keeping a positive attitude, has to help. I don't want to feel bad so I do things to keep myself busy; it is too easy to be home and rest and feel badly.

After packing and visiting I watched a TLC baby show and got some rest. It is nice not to have too many visitors so I don't feel I have to entertain and I can rest when I need and want. I was still feeling hungry so Bob went to the THISTLE to get take out fish and chips. I felt like fish but didn't feel like cooking. Zack was home for dinner and he loves his fish too. I went to bed early and enjoyed a night of TV while Bob went to Wade Currie's stag. He needs to get out and I want to keep the activity as normal as we can.

This is a difficult time for Bob so I want him surrounded by his friends; the young ex-students and athletes at Nelson have kept him close so it does him good to get out. They always ask about me and have been an amazing support through this whole thing.

April 25th - Body a little achy and my head and scalp is very sensitive as the hair is falling out rapidly. This is still the most shocking as I feel so old being bald. I feel so revealed, if that makes sense. I have nothing to hide! I needed some fresh air so Bob and I took Sady (our dog) for a walk. I wore a hoodie as I can't get any sun, especially while in chemo. I was light headed so I held Bob's hand.

We are going to see some homes in Waterdown (Ontario) today. A huge storm in the area but we were still able to see a great home on the 5th Concession. Liz, our realtor, is looking into it since we had some questions with the well and other country concerns. We may consider an offer! We had planned to go to a friend's 50th birthday surprise party but I am tired and Bob would prefer to go with me. My body is sore and muscles ache and my scalp is so sensitive and sore and the hair is now falling out in clumps. I am sad. I have put more of this hair in the same envelope JoAnne and I decided on when it first started falling out.

April 26th - SLOW moving - nauseous, real sick so I had to take the extra ORANGE pill for nausea. Let's see how it works, if it works. I have stayed away from these as I don't like all the medications. I have been taking ginger and ginger ale when feeling nauseous and that has worked up until now. I will not vomit so I will get fresh air or put cold cloths on me before I give in to vomiting.

I wanted to eat and felt like eggs, so Bob made us soft boiled eggs in a cup with toast for dipping. I have always liked these; it is the comfort food you turn to when you are not well. I had breakfast in bed as my head was sore; my hair was falling out and I was tired. I got up about 11 am and made pancakes for lunch. Still have a good appetite. I look for a movie to watch on the Women's channel as I feel it is a stay in and be comfy movie day. These are usually good days unless I feel sick. Some friends came by to visit and Bob drove to Brampton to pick up our taxes from our accountant.

Bob wants to go to Guelph later today to meet a male German shepherd to stud our female Sady with as she will be in heat soon. We want to keep everything normal around here and puppies are part of that plan for the summer. I called Zack to bring me home some ice cream as I had a craving: I like Dairy Queen vanilla cone with chocolate sauce.

I watched more TV and Brock came to visit about 5 pm. He is bringing Thai food for dinner. I have lucked out today with all my cravings and food options. My children have been so good and will do anything I ask. I don't ask for much – after all, how do you say NO to your Mom with cancer, bald and feeling weak and sick.

The books fail to tell you how sore the scalp and head can be when the hair is falling out. Take advantage of the soft baby wool caps the volunteers at the cancer clinic make for sleeping as you need these to sleep - your head hurts just resting against the pillow. This is painful and uncomfortable. Had a hot bath and went to bed early.

April 27th - Spoke with Lois this morning and I can't wait to see her as she has returned from Florida; she lives in Port Credit for the spring and summer months. My temperature is 96.9. We track that too but I forget to note it as I should. Oriol came over at 8:15 am for injection and I got dressed for work.

I worked until 3 pm as I was tired. Lois came over with her dachshund Lily and she brought all my new head covers from the Dallas store. I was so excited to receive these as I need them as my hair is patchy and Brock will shave it all this week.

My body is sore and achy and my temperature is now 98.1. Oriol keeps an eye on my temperature as they are concerned with fever and infection.

April 28th – 4 am, Oriol must come over as she is working an odd shift and I need my injection. My temperature is 97. Got to work about 9:30 am and had a good day at work. I had a good laugh with Jon as we agreed I am still ROCK SOLID despite my chemo treatment and meds as I am completing my work tasks well. The cancer has not disrupted my work. We see the new house at 4 pm as we have had to secure an offer.

Jamie and a few friends came over to watch American Idol but they left about 9 pm as I was tired. Nat is driving from Ottawa and got in about 9:30 pm. She was shocked and disturbed over my hair loss. We chatted for a bit and it feels so good and comforting to have her home. I miss her since she's gone back to school. I know it is tough for her to be away too, but it has to be this way.

April 29th - My scalp is very sore and red. It is ugly and hair groups are in patches so I called Brock and asked if he could shave it soon. Good work day and eventful. My colleagues and others are very complimentary of my scarfs and cancer turbans. Bob met the contractor at the house and we agree to confirm the offer. I went to Brock's salon with Natalie at 5:30 pm since Brock said it would be less busy at the end of the day. The salon was busy but we went to the back of the salon for some privacy and Brock started shaving it. We shed a little tear but it was ok! Empowering as I needed to take some level of control—the little I could have at this time with this disease. Brock ordered me some natural scalp treatment to relieve the soreness and moisturize it. Everyone is the salon was supportive and very kind and wished me well. They all agreed I had a nice shaped head to be bald with no moles or scars. Bob and Zack did not respond well to the baldness and prefer I wear a cap or something. I understand but they need to let me be comfortable and choose what makes me comfortable as the caps hurt at the beginning as the scalp is tender. A bare scalp feels good in the wind or in a cool place so they better get used to it as summer is coming and the warmer weather. I am hot flashing too, as I have been thrown into menopause so a hat will not be happening when I am hot! This is where those cool gels come in handy. (Arbonne detox sea source gelee.)

At 8:30 pm our real estate agent presented the offer and we are excited about it. I am excited too that I have my Mint Chocolate Chip ice cream, which is my special craving right now.

This week, I also noticed no hair growing on my legs – weird! Nice for the upcoming summer and not having to shave. Losing some pubic hair and seem to have no hair under my right arm pit where breast was removed. Lashes and eyebrows still there but I understand they may go or thin out.

April 30th - Slow moving this morning. Tired and nauseous so I went back to bed at 8 am. Oriol came over for my injection and I showered and took my time to get to the office. Arrived about 10 am and was busy all day. This is a great distraction and feels good to be around people and be busy. I left early to meet the inspector at the new house at 4:30 pm. Had a raging headache and it was intolerable during the inspection so I left. Natalie had made dinner so I ate it quick and went to bed. The pain in my head was unbearable and I had never experienced this before. I had taken extra strength Tylenol earlier but I needed something stronger. I had some facial pain and my throat was sore. I was a mess and became afraid. Cool cloths on my head and face were not helping and I had taken more Tylenol too but nothing was working. This was the roughest night yet and just wanted this to be over. I will ask Dr. Tozer about this at my appointment this upcoming Tuesday.

May 1st - Wendy and Helen, friends from work, were coming at noon today and I was hoping I would be OK as I didn't want to cancel. I was so looking forward to seeing them as I really miss them - Wendy especially as we had spent more time together since we left our office in the Guelph area.

I felt well enough to have lunch and really needed it, and we had a great time. We didn't have a long lunch as we had in the past as my body started to spasm and my legs were cramping and tight. That is the best way to describe what a diseased body does during chemotherapy.

Barb R. was also dropping by as she was visiting from up north and she came about 3 pm. Busy day with friends but enjoyed the company.

Mom and Stacey made pork chops and potatos and vegetables and surprised us with it about 5 pm. How thoughtful and appreciated as I had no interest in cooking. Barb was leaving as Mom arrived so they had a short visit too. We had our agent over briefly as we had to sign the offer over again as the terms changed. We were OK with the changes though, and would have a new home – good thing since we had to be out the end of the month!

It is 9:30 pm and my mouth is so dry and my throat is sore and my muscles are all cramped. I am going into a long, hot bath and wish to be left alone. Sometimes I put my candles and stereo in the bathroom and could bathe for an hour or more. It is where I found calm, and the bath made my body stop hurting for a short time. Temporary relief was good and I looked forward to my baths. I noticed some pieces of hair in the tub afterwards when cleaning the tub. It must be from my pubic area or head as there isn't much anywhere else. Some lashes maybe as they were starting to get thin. I took a sleeping pill tonight; a stronger one as I was hurting and anxious - we hadn't back from their agent as he was out of town. I wanted this home all signed and sealed and deal closed. I hope tomorrow brings about a better day as it's the weekend.

May 2nd- By 10 am we heard that our offer was accepted and all is firm! Paula H. came over for a visit and brought me a beautiful soft chemo blanket her niece knit for me. It was baby soft and in shades of greys and blues – love it and so comforting and practical. My friends thought of the best gifts! I have taken note as I now know what the best gifts are as I struggled with what to give someone who was ill. What could they find useful? My friends have given me the best ideas and the most generous gifts. She also gave me a soft wool cap for my head; your scalp hurts on the pillow and you need something to wear initially until your scalp is less sensitive. The cancer clinics offer you bins of caps that volunteers have made. Pick the softest ones and pick a few. Don't feel you are being greedy or rude to take more than one. I wish I had taken more at the time.

Patti from the curling club dropped by to say hello and brought me some lovely baked goods. She also delivered some healing CD's from Linda, another fellow curler, which was nice. Patti offered to do any Neupogen injections if Oriol couldn't as Patti is a nurse too. Very thoughtful again. I am so blessed to have such amazing people in my life.

Brock and I are going shopping to Buffalo tomorrow for a little outing; he knows I like my US shopping, as does he. I have to take the extra strength Tylenol every 6 hours for the body jerks and cramping. Purchased more Tylenol in the US as it is less expensive, as is the Biotene for my mouth soreness.

May 3rd - Brock over bright and early and we were off to Buffalo by 9 am. Brock drove his new car, a "GOLF", to the US and was thrilled I went on the first long drive with him. We had a great time and successful shopping trip. I bought some more appropriate tops as I had my new disfigured chest I wanted to bring less attention to, so he helped me purchase looser fitting tops with some scarf like accessories on the chest to hide the right side.

We did our quick TOPS and BEER shop and headed home. They recognized me as a chemo patient with my cap on and such a white drawn face with little brows and lashes. They were so sensitive and kind and asked me nothing as they usually do. I was shocked as we usually get asked so many questions and may even get asked to pull over to be searched or pay duty. I must go over more often with my cap on or use them even when I am healed if this works like this!

Mom and Dad came to dinner at 5 pm. for a barbecue and got a good laugh at my cap and border story. I made some great ribs for dinner and surprised myself as I am not a good rib maker. I had a bath and was in bed by 7 pm. My family and friends do not expect any late nights or entertainment lately as they know how tired I am and are so accommodating. Even with a sleeping pill, I only get 3-4 hours of good sleep. Start to fuss and toss and turn after 4 am.

May 4th - Bob says I am snoring more so he thinks I am sleeping better. I know I am restless. My GP tells me the sleeping pill does cause snoring. That makes sense as I didn't snore before. I worked from 9-2 today and felt a little better. The skin on my scalp feels better so the creams do work. Make sure you use a safe cream with no chemicals or mineral oil. I had my appointment with Dr. Tozer and nurse Leslie reviewed my file. I weighed in at 128 which seemed high but I did have heavy sandals on. I had been losing weight as you do during chemo. She explained thoroughly the next round of the T in ACT treatment, the TAXOL mix. This would be a longer treatment, more muscle pain expected but less nauseous. She explained it may go an hour longer so they put in the bed rather than the chair if you wish to rest or lay out and be more comfortable. Had bloodwork to make sure we are on for tomorrow and will see Dr. Tozer tomorrow too before chemo.

May 5th - Met with Dr. Tozer and reviewed the first rounds of chemo. The best part of the meeting was that he agreed to order a nurse to come to our new home in Waterdown to do the Neupogen injections. I had become so anxious about these and Bob could not do them and neither could I. Some people do their own but we are not needle people. The last time we tried Bob stabbed me like it was and EPI pen and it hurt! He is not comfortable trying—we did try several times on fruit and just couldn't get it right. Dr. Tozer agreed that I shouldn't feel anxiety about this so he will make the referral. Quiet evening and watched American Idol. Uneventful night and a bit anxious for new chemo tomorrow.

May 6th - Did some shopping and banking before chemo today. Cathy G. is my chemo partner today which is so nice. We went out to lunch at 11 am as my chemo was set for 1 pm today. I had requested mornings but it was later this time. Tough day as the head rush came on strong after this Taxol injection. As I drove home, my head got worse so I was pleased she was driving with me. By 4:30 pm the headache was unbearable. I went straight to bed and took more Tylenol and cold cloths on my head. I got up about 8 pm and had some dinner, as you must eat. I felt better standing up or sitting and not laying down so I sat up for the rest of the evening.

I went to bed as I was tired but slept laying up as I watched some TV. The pain got worse so more Tylenol and more cold cloths. I had trouble sleeping and was up at 1 am and went to the spare bedroom to sleep as I was disrupting Bob and he needed to sleep too. Took some nausea meds so it had to be bad; I don't like those as they tend to constipate me. I prefer to take more natural remedies for nausea like ginger or cold towels or go into a cold space or use cool gel. Now they have chew candy to help during chemo.

May 7th - Did some work on the home computer as I was up early and could not sleep. Katy, our mortgage girl, said appraisal went well and all conditions can be removed as financing all approved. Had a quiet day of rest and did some packing with Natalie in the afternoon. I love having Natalie around as I missed her while at school in Ottawa. My children prepared a nice barbecue and we had a great evening. I love being around the children and their friends. It makes such a difference and makes things feel normal. We watched Grey's Anatomy and then I had to go to bed. Real tired.

May 8th - I had a better sleep, about 6 hours consistently. Did some very light housework and waited for Oriol to come give me my injection. Took more nausea pills as I had to get some packing done and I knew day 2 after chemo I would start feeling sick. It is so predictable and that is why I like chemo on a Wednesday so I can get sick over the weekend and feel OK for work on Monday.

Victoria popped by today and I was exhausted by 4 pm when she left. My eyes are sore and dry so the Dr. suggested Natural Tears and they seem to work. This can be a side effect too. Had some pain and tenderness in my head and neck so I took my sleeping pills early and went to bed.

Shoulder blades real sore so I took Tylenol and will look into massage. Cymbalta helps with joint pain too I am told. I spent most of the day in bed watching the Women's Channel. I watched Stepmom, of all movies I could choose. How provocative and sad. I cried but I think I needed a good cry. I felt hot all day so this must be the menopause creeping up; they said this would happen. My head and face burns so I guess these are the bad menopausal hot flashes!

It is Mother's Day and Natalie brings me a beautiful plant and an emotional card that had me crying again. Lots of sobbing these days but I think this is all part of it. Had another long bath and gave myself a lovely scalp treatment which felt wonderful!

I made dinner for Bob and myself—which isn't right on Mother's Day but OK I guess as I owe him many dinners. Tomorrow we take our dog Sady to the stud in Arthur (we breed German Shepherds) so that will be a nice Sunday drive. I notice red and purple dots on the tops of my legs but nowhere else. Another side effect I read about somewhere. I spoke to Marie, Jeanne's mom, on the phone (she is in BC) and we had some great laughs! You need to laugh and everyone needs a refreshing Marie!

May 14th - Fairly good week and kids all came around for Mother's Day eventually. Oriol coming every morning for injections and she notices the rash too but said it is normal. Body feeling tighter and took Imodium for diarrhea. Appetite good but nauseous. Stomach cramps so this must be the Taxol chemo as I didn't feel this with the first AC rounds.

May 15th - Cathy F. from the curling club is coming over and we are going for a pedicure and lunch. I am so excited to go out with her. I even had a glass of wine and I hadn't had one since the day before my mastectomy (3 months). It tasted great! We had a terrific day and caught up and she had me home about 2 pm as I was tired and I wanted to prepare for our garage sale tomorrow. Was in bed by 10 pm but watched the Farrah Fawcett special – her battle she lost with cancer. Wrong show to watch but interesting. Learned much and needed to see a REAL story.

May 16th & 17th - The weekend was busy and garage sale was a success. We got rid of much stuff and felt more organized for the move. I visited a friend and neighbor who had just completed her chemotherapy and radiation for colon cancer so we shared our story and it felt good and very helpful to know someone else understands and gets what you are going through.

May 18th - Victoria Day holiday. Many visitors and loads of fun and activity but very tiring! Need a good sleep as I have computer maintenance tomorrow at work and appointment with Dr. Tozer for bloodwork.

May 19th - Chemo again tomorrow so blood taken today to ensure all is ok with blood count. Dr. Gudelis, or Dr. Susan as I call her, saw me and gave me new prescriptions for meds. She suggests I combine Adavan with the Zoplicone sleeping pill as that may give me better sleep. She gave me Tylenol with codeine for the body pain as she feels it may get worse with more chemo.

May 20th - Chemo day! Deb McMillan, Kyle's mom coming today. I had a few hours at work this morning and arrived home at noon so Deb could drive us to our chemo appointment. We waited until 2:40 pm in the chemo lounge to get in. Joy Dooley was there and felt bad that we waited so long. Joy was my friend (also the nurse who did the orientation) and was shocked to see me in the group. It is nice to have her there as she provides a comfort and familiarity. Anna was a new nurse and she wasn't having a good day. She stuck the IV in and it hurt! It stung and wasn't where my needle usually goes in. She put it in my arm where they take blood and I never have the chemo needle there. She knew I was not happy and suggested another location for the IV and perhaps another nurse. Bev took over who I had seen before and she was much happier and so gentle. Nurses can have bad days too! Bev administered the chemo and sat with us for a bit.

Deb had packed treats for us and we had a great time and Joy came by too! The head rush happened again but it wasn't as bad as 2 weeks ago. I had taken the Tylenol just in case it got worse. On the way home, Deb and I bought some lotto tickets as we felt we needed something GOOD to happen in our lives.

May 23rd - Predictable days after chemo. Feeling sick so stayed in bed most of the day watching my TV. Took Tylenol, anti-nausea meds - took them all! Took stool softeners and Senokot as I knew this was going to constipate me but I needed relief! Rough couple of days!

My Dad's birthday was the 23rd but I felt so poor I didn't do anything for him. I was cramped, sick, and nauseous and wanted to see no one. Took many baths and took sleeping pills and tried to go to bed early.

May 24th - This day was even worse! Nothing seems to help but I am sick of being sick and being in bed so I want to go out and see people and take part in Kyle McMillan's fundraising event and watch the football. I need to be around good people and FUN! My children were participating as were many of our friends. I wanted to show my support for and contribute to the fundraising event and their Ride to Conquer Cancer, in his memory.

Saw JoAnne and Matt, Elaine and Cathy. They were volunteering at the BBQ so I stayed under the tent in the shade with them. I think people like to see me as they are uncertain about how I may be responding to treatment and coping so it is refreshing and a relief to know I am OK.

We stayed for an hour and took part in the festivities. It was good to see the McMillans and all the other Nelson ex-students and families who were involved with the fundraiser – they are such tremendous supporters and friends of the McMillans and were committed to the events in Kyle's memory. A quiet evening after that day outing.

May 25th - BIG CONSTIPATION despite all the stool softeners and Senokot I am taking. PAIN like I have never felt. In tears as I am in so much discomfort. So bad I called Dr. Tozer's office - Leslie explained it would eventually pass and to be patient and let the meds work. (Easy for her to say.) Struggled in pain and discomfort all day. It got so bad that I needed to get out and move around so I went to work for a few hours in the late afternoon. I usually was able to return to work on the Monday after the Wed. chemo but couldn't this morning as the pain was too much. The evening was tough with a sore back and sore butt as I had not had a bowel movement. Nauseous too so a miserable night. Abdominal cramps and poor sleep.

May 26th - Tired after a rough night but I wanted to work as the Directors were meeting with the Head Office Marketing Director to discuss the Golden Horseshoe conference I was overseeing. I was worried I would have to leave the meeting suddenly if I felt a bowel movement coming on or had the 'runs' as a result of the stool softeners. I struggled through that meeting but did it. A small movement (that I had been waiting for and had worried about) came after the meeting. I was nauseous and grey and the girls at the office were concerned about me as I was struggling and my color worried them. I had to go home and they didn't like me driving but I had no choice as I needed to get home and be in my own bathroom. This was 2 pm.

I drove home somehow and by 3:30 I was curled over in pain with terrible cramps. I had very loose diarrhea and was so pleased to be in my own home in my own bathroom in my own loose pyjamas. We all feel like this when we are sick. My butt and back were so sore and I had never felt pain like this, not even at childbirth! Now I know the pain people talk about when they talk constipation – OUCH!

As the evening went on, the pain increased as the bowel movements did but I knew this had to happen to get rid of this incredible pain. I will not take any more Tylenol with codeine as this has caused it. On the toilet much through the evening and more cramps and a real sore ass! Took sleeping pill but was up at 3 and 5 am to use the bathroom.

May 27th - Could not go to work after the night I had. Needed a day in bed and to heal and rest. Called Jon at 5 am when I was up and told him I wouldn't be in. He has been wonderful and never makes me feel bad for taking the time off. I did some work emails but was in bed most of the day. Someone had suggested a citrus facial for my head pain, so I tried it and it felt great. I don't want to take meds for the headaches as I afraid of constipation so this facial and oils are a healthier, holistic option.

Approaching Sunrise

JoAnne Porter called and we suddenly made a spontaneous plan - those are always the best - to go to the spa and go out for dinner. She had a pedicure while I had my facial so that was fun. We went to dinner on Brant Street at some new trendy spot, and it was a great time out! We all need to do more of that, especially when we are having a difficult time. Late night for me as we got home just after 8 pm. My headache was still there but she took my mind off it and I didn't think about it while out enjoying my day and evening with her. Had a bath and off to bed at 9 with much needed sleeping pill.

May 28th - Slow moving but got to work by 9:30 am. Busy day and worked until 3:45. An eventful, good day of work, which I need to keep my mind busy. I need another more positive focus. I rested for an hour as Natalie was taking me to Jamie's mom's home to attend Lois' jewelry party. It was fun to see everyone as it was mostly family and good friends. I was home by 9:30 and to bed by 10.

I am just starting to be regular again and having normal bowel movements – what a relief! I still have the headaches so I think I will use more oils and cool cloths and no meds.

My neighbour Oriol did my last Neupogen injection today. She commented on how good my skin is as I don't have the brown and purple colored rash and marks from the injections. She thought my skin looked better. Could it be the facial I had?

May 29th - Woke with a runny nose and sore throat so didn't try to go to work. I listen to my body when it feels weak and I felt I needed a day of rest. Bad metal taste in my mouth today that I thought I tasted a bit earlier in the week too. I have been rinsing and brushing with the Biotene 4-6 times daily as I am so worried to get any mouth sores. Really don't like this metal taste, and I can't recall why they say this happens.

Have hemorrhoids now from the past bowel issues so using Anusol. They are sore too but I have had these at childbirth so I feel OK with these as I know they go away with TUCK pads and Anusol cream.

Terri M. called and we planned to get together soon with the curling girls. They have all called and written on my care page and sent treats. I am so lucky to have these amazing ladies in my life.

Did some more packing and sorting and all the kids were here for dinner which was nice. In bed by 9 pm.

May 30th & May 31st - I needed to get out so Bob and I went for a walk. Need to exercise and be outdoors. Plan to get my prosthetic bra today from Julie D. Have a few mouth sores; I keep rinsing with the Biotene and flossing more than usual as I am obsessed with my mouth and cannot handle sores. Need to eat less spice, more yogurt, more fibre and be so careful to prevent these mouth sores. I am rinsing with salt water and probably overdoing it! I am staying on top of the constipation and keeping away from more codeine and continuing the Senokot and stool softeners. I will ask Dr. Tozer about Percocet or Senaten to try to use something else for the head pain after the chemo. I see Dr. Tozer June 2nd so I will make note of that.

I went out with JoAnne P. to get some new furniture for the new house. She and I have a great time and many laughs.

The writing in my journal was bad so I imagine I was on a lot of medication throughout that weekend.

June 1st - Much better day, thank God! I wrote on my site that I am thrilled to be into June as that means we are closer to this being over! Great day at work and good evening packing and eating stir fry amongst boxes and packing equipment. Natalie and I went to visit Patti and Jacklyn and we had some good laughs. Great to catch up; we hadn't seen one another for a while since the girls aren't playing basketball together anymore.

June 2nd - Work at 9 am and off to see the doctors for 10:30 am. Waited a long time as they were busy. I was down 2 lbs and took the anti-nausea meds that I take now the day before my chemo. Let's hope this helps! Saw the new nurse Nancy and she was great. They are all good and thorough. She told me that my period may return after chemo. This was news to me as I thought the chemo caused menopause and you can't have periods. I guess we will see as that was a bonus to the cancer. She agreed the codeine caused the constipation, but sometimes you need the codeine. Taxol can cause more leg pain and soreness but other patients suggest it will get less as the chemo finishes. Let's hope so! Went back to work and had an appointment to get my new prosthetic form and the new bra from Greta's Flair. Julie took great care of me: she did all the paperwork and faxed it in, as some payment is covered. I had a quiet night and was anxious for chemo tomorrow.

June 3rd - Did not sleep well. Mom and Dad picked me up at 8:15 am for 9 am chemo. It was my parents' turn - Bob would come in the afternoon to pick me up, as he had not been yet. Bob didn't wish to come as he doesn't like hospitals and especially the chemo unit. I had no reaction today and all went well which my parents were relieved to see. They left about noon as Bob was coming soon. I was tired and wanted to rest. I had my TV on and was into one of the talk shows when Jan C. came by to visit, which was nice. Her son played basketball with Zack and she works at the clinic so it was nice to see her. Bob and I left about 2. Only 3 more chemotherapy sessions left!

June 4th - Less nauseous and not much of a headache so the pills taken the day before did work. Lower back pain and leg cramping but tolerable. Kathy M. dropped by while nurse Marg there and we all had a nice visit. I will miss these visits with Marg when we move next week.

Everyone likes my new fake boob. It looks real but it is heavy and hard. I hate putting it in and out of the bra and into its little case. It is like a mini hat case but keeps it clean and safe. At 400 dollars, I will place it in a safe place!

June 5th & 6th - Did some errands over the weekend. Replied to personal emails that I hadn't done for a while and then Oriol came over for my injection – sometimes I have them at night now. Meeting John and Karen at the Keg tonight for dinner which will be nice. I am looking forward to a big steak! And red wine!

June 7th - ACHY! Very tired and watching the Women's channel again – sappy, love stories so I must be a little down. I may go for a hot tub as the jets go directly on my legs and help the aches and pains. Took some meds and ginger for the nausea. Bad night and irritable. Woke at 8 pm, very uncomfortable, sweaty, miserable and in unbearable pain! Popped some more Tylenol with codeine as I had no choice. Ugly night!

June 8th - Slow moving and very tired. Oriol called me at 8:15 am and asked me to come to her home next door for my injection. I came home and showered and was off to work by 9:30 am.

Very busy at the office which makes by day go by faster and keep my mind off all these aches and discomfort. I was home by 4 pm. Work distracts me from the illness and treatments so I like going each day, despite how tired I am at the end of the day. Natalie made a lovely dinner and my parents came over to join us.

I had to have a hot tub as my body ached so badly. I position myself right at the jets to get the strength of the water on the specific areas that hurt. It does help. I watched the Bachelorette and enjoyed banana and chocolate popsicles to soothe my mouth; I feel a sore coming on and the cold seems to help - or at least I think it does. I am still so paranoid of a mouth sore and will do anything to prevent one.

June 9th - I worked until 1:45 pm as I had an appointment with Dr. Kym, the radiation oncologist. I saw him at 2:20 and he explained radiation – why, how, effects, outcomes and the chance of cancer re-occurrence. It was a little discouraging as he was brutally honest which I was appreciative of. Still, his explanation of my cancer being "borderline and aggressive" rattled me and he explained that this is why my radiation was going to be intense. He spoke of how it could reoccur and what is typical with my form of cancer. I do want all my physicians to be honest but even so I wasn't prepared to hear it - I had been feeling so positive!

Given how well I have done, my attitude, energy and general health, he he told me I should be OK. This made me feel better.

He is setting up the appointment for tattoos and CAT scan for the radiation. It will be 25 sessions daily for 6 weeks. He suggested "down time" and R&R – yeah right. Dr. Kym was very clear explaining the area that would be involved, - the breast, under arm, arm pit, shoulder and neck. Again, he stressed the size, depth and spreading of the cancer. I get it! It was bad! They have to tell you everything and I am OK with that. I do tune some of it out as you have to and you tend to, as it is much to grasp. I should have had someone with me to hear all of that!

Did groceries on the way home and bath and bed by 8 pm.

June 10th - Great work day and less pain and body soreness. Did some packing tonight as I was feeling better. Jon away at conference so week is busy! Working full days Thursday and Friday in Jon's absence. Jon returned after 10 am Friday and we reviewed the conference he attended. Fairly good week for me!

June 13th - Great day packing house and running errands. Felt pretty good and kept busy, which helps as it keeps your mind off the aches and bad stuff!

June 14th - So tired given the past few days and week. Bob and Zack took 2 big trailer loads to the new house. I laid low as I was tired. I cleaned out the refrigerator and freezers. Needed some alone time too!

June 15th - My family all chipping in to sort and clear house with me as it's MOVING DAY! I have the conference in Niagara tomorrow and this is chemo week so I have to go to work. I am so excited to pick up JACK LENGYEL, my guest speaker, from the Buffalo airport. Bob and I are so thrilled to meet him and spend time with him. He is the coach who the movie WE ARE MARSHALL was written about. Matthew McConaughey played Jack. The movie was released in 2006, just 3 years ago. I called him directly instead of going through his agent since I heard that a while ago he had done an amazing event at Wilfred Laurier. I knew this man, this COACH, would appeal to my group; a group full of men and women who would appreciate his gift, his spirit, his coaching, his beliefs and his inspiration and leadership.

When I started communicating with Jack, I had to make him aware of my cancer and tell him I would miss his speech at the conference I was overseeing as I had chemo sessions. He remains one of the most powerful and inspirational people who touched me and influenced me during this time and this journey. I was meant to meet him along the way in this journey. I was blessed to have this man's wisdom and hope smother me in the few days we spent together.

My chemo falls on the first day of the conference so Bob is picking Jack up with me - Bob is so pumped to meet this coaching legend and movie hero! I have planned to meet Jack after the conference as I have arranged for him to speak at the Hamilton Sport Volunteer Awards 2 days later. I planned this with our business and community partners at the City of Hamilton when I knew the conference and the awards were being held in the same week. Couldn't have picked a better speaker for both events!

We were thrilled, as were the conference attendees and all participants at the Sports Awards. This man is a true legend. When he asked for the position of Coach of the Marshall Football team back in 1971, after they lost 75 football players, staff and coaches, he said, "I knew this was a chance for me to give back; I was their last choice and their only choice... This is about everything football stands for – not giving up, perseverance and sportsmanship. This isn't the Jack Lengyel story. It's about Huntington, West Virginia and Marshall University. It's about hope, faith and loyalty and the values of a community....When I got there, I thought I was rebuilding a football team, I guess I found out it was much more than that."

This is just a NUGGET from the many words and many things I took from the movie, and of course most importantly from him personally. He continues to contact us and he has a very special place in my journey and my heart.

June 16th - After doing all my blood work and meeting with Dr. Tozer to re-view my tests and know everything was OK for chemo, we were on our way to meet Jack in Buffalo and get him to my conference in Niagara Falls. We recognized him immediately from the movie and his many media pieces. On the car ride to Niagara Falls (Canada), we were overwhelmed with his character and passionate stories. He went on and on as we asked questions; we were star-struck and amazed by his genuine nature and simplicity. Bob and he spoke about the Dallas Cowboys and past coaches as Jack knows them all well; he shared tale after tale of the NFL greats keeping Bob enter-tained and hanging on Jack's every word.

This drive and dinner to the conference hotel had to be one of the most enjoyable and inspirational experiences ever! In such a short time, he made me feel like I had known him for much longer – amazing that from this initial meeting he would remain a close person to both Bob and me. You don't get this feeling this quickly from many people. Jack is a remarkable man, and he left something so valuable to both of us that it is hard to put into words.

The conference went well without me – of course I called in a few times to make sure all went well and Jack was taken care of. My colleagues took good care of him, and I even asked of few of my special friends to drive back with Jack to Hamilton so they could share the type of experience Bob and I did.

June 17th - Lois came to the house the next day to pick me up for chemo; she has wanted to come from the beginning, and this was her date. She and I had SO much catching up to do! We arrived at 8:50 am.

I don't know if I could have handled all this without Lois. She has been there for me since the beginning and has been my rock. She knows what to say, when to say it and how. She is brilliant and the most amazing and generous friend. Lois flew back from Florida when I was diagnosed, appeared during the "Bandage ceremony", called me once or more each day thinking and doing all the things I forgot or need to do. This is RAW, REAL friendship and I am blessed to have her in my life!

She had been on an Alaskan cruise for 2 weeks with her family so we really did have much to catch up on. We have never gone that long without speaking, NEVER.

She sat with me and watched the IV, the chemo, and we chatted and snacked on healthy treats. She has always been healthy and lives very healthy. She made me comfortable and fed the parking meter during the chemo. We had about 30 minutes left in my chemo Taxol drip when a patient across the hall had a bad reaction to her chemo. All the bells and lights were flashing and all the staff ran to her bed, closing the drapes around her. They warn you at your first chemo session that this may happen; this is why they stay close during the first chemo treatment. This was frightening; it is easy for PANIC to take over in the chemo suite. It wasn't the normal thing though - it is usually calm and quiet while everyone is receiving treatment. After 20 minutes, they told everyone that she was OK and being monitored more closely.

It was around this time that Lois gave me a special gift that I wear to this day, and now have given to many others. I have a thick silver band on my 4th finger on my right hand with the words inscribed, "What cancer cannot do....steal eternal life, conquer the spirit, suppress memories, kill friendship, cripple love, corrode faith, shatter hope, destroy peace, silence courage, invade the soul."

I don't how many times I have read and reread and referred to these words and found it empowering and true!

June 18th- My colleagues were so pleased with the conference I had planned and especially thrilled with Jack's presentation. My friend Jay who drove Jack back to Hamilton was so pleased I had asked him to accompany Jack – he told me that it was a memorable drive, as was ours that day from the airport.

June 19th - Like most days after chemo, I was aching and in pain. The achiness gets worse as chemo progresses so now on Tylenol 4 times a day. Legs and hands tingly and starting to numb. I will start using the cold mitts and boots to avoid this neuropathy (a friend told me about this).

June 20th - Spent most of the day in bed and completed my memory book for Lois' 50th birthday party. I have a box with photos so I am doing it now before the box is misplaced at the new house.

June 21st (Father's Day) - Not well. My new nurse Wilma starts today. Very little to say; we don't chat the way Marg and I did. She does the injection and leaves. I miss Marg but I knew I had to change nurses as I am moving to a new community and region. All overseen by CCAC. I know Marg will come see me.

June 22nd - Good but long day at work. I have lots to clean up from conference but pleased to hear how all my colleagues enjoyed it. Numbness worse in hands and feet. MOVED into new home later in afternoon. I couldn't do any lifting so I didn't go to the house this morning. Air conditioning not installed yet so it is HOT! Not good for me and my joints! Humidity and dampness affects the joints.

June 23th - Not feeling well so only worked from 9-1. Nauseous and feel weird. Body tingling.

June 24th-26th- Went to work and then stayed with parents - they have air conditioning! Need to sleep better so I will stay there until our new home has air conditioner and is somewhat organized. I can't handle the craziness of the move. Returned to new house on evening of 26th (Friday) and did some sorting and unpacking: Bob, Zack and Jamie other family members did most of it. I have no patience to deal with servicemen and cable people. Bob came home earlier to deal with it all.

June 27th - Achy and agitated! Frustrated as I am not well enough to organize house. Have to accept it and let others do it! I have no energy or care to do anything which is so unlike me!

June 28th - Quiet - all the STACEY men were at our family golf tournament, leaving just Nat and I at the house. She and I did errands and went out to have Thai food for dinner.

June 29th - Very busy day at work as my IG golf tournament is fast approaching. I am focused on this so it keeps me busy and on task. I am easily distracted these days so this focus is good and much needed. Even therapeutic. Worked full day until 5. Felt pretty good.

June 30th - Lab work at 8:45 and appointment with Dr. Tozer to review things. Got to work at 11 am and was busy until 6 pm. My fingers were tingly and numb and I felt some difficulty holding cups and writing.

July 1st - Canada Day! The show must go on! I am trying so hard to keep life normal and celebrate the normal holidays and special occasions. Our family is close and gets together with friends and in-laws for most events. An outcome of all of this is that I have lost weight, so I was excited to fit into an old Canada T-shirt (size 6) for our outing to Jamie's family party! Everyone was very sensitive to me and I met one of Jamie's neighbors, which was very encouraging. She is also a survivor and she lives life to its fullest, not letting cancer disrupt her life.

July 2nd – Second Last Chemo! Mom and Dad had been wanting to take me to chemo again so this was their next date. This was one of the longer sessions, so, like the first time, we arranged for them to take me and Bob to pick me up - Bob had still been avoiding this since he hates hospitals. I hoped it went as smoothly as the first time they took me - Mom only had radiation years ago, not chemo, and no parent likes to see their child hurt.

My Dad is very protective and hates that he can't control this disease for me and take the pain away. This is something no one has control of and that is the MOST difficult thing. We waited for 30 minutes so they saw many different patients in and out of the chemo suites. They experienced the comfort and "family feel" here, the "we are all in this together" approach. Many of us know one another as we have endured treatment together and know one another's families and friends.

This is a huge comfort and the volunteers go out of their way to make sure you are comfortable, offering juices and treats - sometimes the therapy dogs come to visit, which is so calming and so appreciated! They are usually labs or retrievers. This is part of the healing journey!

It took the nurse today 2 nasty attempts to get the IV in which never happens. Some do it better than others and you learn quickly who your favourite nurses are. Dad didn't like seeing me uncomfortable as this hurt today as they continued to poke to get the IV in place. Mom shows little emotion as I have suggested earlier in the book.

We chatted until 11 am when "The View" (TV talk show) came on and I wanted to watch it to fall asleep. Every chemo bed or chair has a TV so you can bring your ear plugs and enjoy. As this chemo is the 5 hour Taxol one, I usually take a little nap. This was the time for Mom and Dad to leave; it was enough for them and they knew I needed to rest and wasn't feeling well.

I INSISTED the nurse get me the COOL mitts and booties as the numbness or neuropathy was getting worse each chemo treatment. Joy, my nurse who took over (the nurse / friend who did my orientation at the beginning of the book), said nerve damage could be permanent. Bob came about 1:30 pm and waited while they did the rinse, which is the end of the chemo session.

July 3rd – July 5th - Uneventful and quiet after chemo. When I wasn't resting I was sorting through boxes and trying to get organized in the new house. I had a headache and was achy. The achiness was normal but the bad headache was new. I thought fresh air would be good, since that usually makes me feel better, so we went to the greenhouse up the street and purchased flowers and shrubs for gardens. Didn't stay too long as my body hurt and I have done too much today. The cool air always makes me feel better and I suggest this to anyone going through this. A cool blast of air conditioning or a cool wind or a cold cloth on your head can help.

July 6th-8th - Very busy few days at work organizing golf tournament and changing and adding late foursomes, collecting prizes and auction items. They were busy, full days but I had Bob helping me – there was no way I could do it alone. The girls at the office helped me with the program and they are a great help! They will volunteer the day of the event as we need all the girls on the holes and assisting with specialty holes and putting contests. This year they are even more helpful; they know I am struggling, especially in this heat! Heat and chemo treatments do not go well together!

Bob and I have made a few trips to Heron Point Golf Club to take prizes and programs, etc. I need to be more organized as my "chemo fog" makes me forget and I am not as sharp these days. They tell you this fog lasts throughout chemo so I am paying extra attention to being organized: I keep a journal and write everything down or include it my tasks on my computer. The golf staff, who I have known for years and consider a few of them my friends, are sad to hear of my cancer and the treatments. They are shocked to see me bald and so thin and drawn.

July 9th – (Tournament Day) - I am tired and overwhelmed but I put my smile on and receive all the clients and colleagues and community partners like I always do. This year I receive extra hugs as they are surprised to hear of my illness and see me as I am. They are all so supportive and concerned, embracing me with so much love. They too are family; I have known some of them for 20 years - as long as Jon and I have been working together.

I could not be in the sun so I stayed inside the clubhouse and set up the auction and prize tables. Great day and event, with an emotional end for me when Jon acknowledged me, and the cancer, and presented me with a huge bouquet of flowers. I received a standing ovation and I looked at Bob and Jon and the tears started. As crazy as my week went, it got crazier - we had planned an Open House at the new house for Saturday! Yes, we are crazy! Cancer makes you a little crazier, and sometimes you need to be, so go with it and have fun!

July 10th - Did some shopping and cleaning for the house party tomorrow.

July 11th - Best Party ever! An early morning in Westdale picking up cake - we were celebrating Lois' and sisters-in-law Vanessa's and Karen's birthdays as well as having a housewarming gathering. Our guests started arriving at 3 pm and the BBQ party was loads of fun. Everyone loved the property and house and had a great time celebrating the birthdays, one another and my recovery! It was hot so the cap came off and I had to be bald - like most of Bob's cousins and my 2 boys! The kids organized a DJ for the evening and he started setting up about 7 - all their friends came over and got the REAL party started.

Life goes on and this cancer hasn't stopped the celebrations and fun. You need to celebrate friends and family and LIFE as you never know what can happen.

July 12th- Lois invited us to her home in Port Credit for her real birthday dinner. We shared a great afternoon, which turned into a bit of a later night with us returning home after 9 pm. I always have cocktails with Nick and Lois so I had a rum and coke and red wine - hoping to sleep well tonight.

July 13th – I am off this week but have to follow up about the golf tournament proceeds and of course there is clean-up work after such an event. Best to work at home with no interruptions. Took a drive to the cottage in Fergus to visit with Mom and Dad and napped all afternoon. The weekend must have taken a great deal out of me!

July 14th – Have lab work done and have appointment to see Dr. Tozer at 9:30 am. I dropped some sponsor posters and the tent from the tournament off at the office and Jon asked me to work for 2 hours. I couldn't believe it, but I stayed since he has done so much for me. He needed to discuss the tournament proceeds, which wasn't surprising since we were always excited with the final number we made for the charity. I was tired so returned home by 3. So excited for my LAST CHEMO tomorrow ! ! ! !

July 15th - LAST CHEMO ! ! ! !

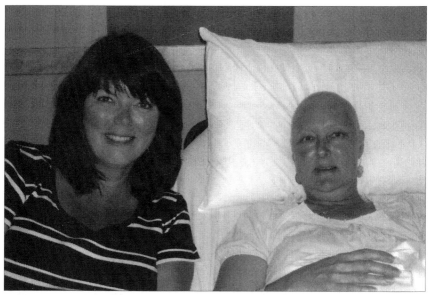

JoAnne Jurus and I during my last chemo treatment.

July 15ᵗʰ continued....JoAnne Jurus (Jon's sister in law) picked me up at 8:40 am to take me to my 9:30 am last chemotherapy treatment. We made a poster with MY LAST CHEMO written on it and we took many photos. We want to send a pic to Good Morning America as they have their 3 simple words promotion on right now and these 3 words on the poster are my very special 3 words! We laughed and carried on and wanted to ring the bell at the end of chemo, but we didn't as I felt guilty rubbing it in for those who may have just started or were struggling with their treatment. I was tired and had a mighty head rush again so we took it slow leaving the cancer clinic. I had one of my favourite nurses too so that was so comforting! I filled all my medications for the next month and will return to the cancer centre next Monday for radiation tattooing. My first tattoo!

July 16ᵗʰ - Did some shopping to finish getting gifts for the Currie wedding, one of Bob's former students.

July 17ᵗʰ - I start feeling achy, as usual, as we approach the weekend. Had a nap before the 4 pm wedding but struggled with what to wear - I need to have a cap to match my dress. This was stressful: I am bald, tired, feel very unattractive and have no idea what to wear to this muggy and humid wedding, especially knowing my body will ache terribly with this weather. I end up wearing a navy cocktail dress with a navy and white bandana. Turned out to be a poor choice as the bandana slips off my head since there is nothing for it to grasp on to.

It was a lovely wedding with fabulous speeches and it was so wonderful to be included. Party started at 7 pm and we left as we wouldn't be dancing and I was exhausted.

July 18ᵗʰ - Lazy Day! Very achy and frustrated. I was in a foul mood so stayed much to myself.

July 19ᵗʰ - Felt terrible: more numbness and pain in legs and hands. Frustrated and miserable. Just tired of being sick and tired! No energy and couldn't complete all the things I needed to do around the new house.

July 20ᵗʰ - I slept until 8 am so I must have needed it. Feeling a little better and I know that rest helps so you must force yourself to get that much needed rest and healing. Listen to your body - it tells you everything. Slow moving but got to work about 10 am. Worked a full day!

I wrote very little the next weeks as I had little to say. I was down and very frustrated. I had very little energy and it took everything in me to get up, dress and go to work. I am exhausted by 5 pm and get ready for bed. I have to move slowly in the morning and stretch to get the body moving as it is stiff and achy always. My right ankle swells and bothers me.

August 2nd - We attended another Nelson alumni wedding, the Behie wedding, and despite how I was feeling it was very enjoyable. Again I struggled with what to wear, but I was better prepared this time with a more appropriate dress and headwear. The dress was more formal so the headpiece looked silly. I would prefer to go bald but this was a posh wedding and felt very formal.

August 5th - I had started taking Tamoxifen, so maybe I am feeling bad because of the new meds. Perhaps the sadness or achiness is a side effect. Let's see how this goes - I need this medication since it is a preventative drug to keep the cancer away! I want it to work. I have little energy for anything but I toughed it out and worked Monday - Thursday while Jon was away. I am slow some mornings but Jon understands and allows me to come into work late when I feel ready. I need to stretch and move before I can get up and moving, shower, etc. If I don't stretch and if I rush in the mornings, I feel sick and crampy. A poor start to the day sets the tone for the entire day and week. I need to move and sitting and resting makes it worse, so work is good! Jon was away for two weeks so I needed to be there. I started REIKI and MASSAGE THERAPY at The Circle of Light, a local naturopathic centre here in Waterdown (Ontario). This place was suggested by a friend – Kim, my therapist, was fabulous and so sensitive to my needs and treatment. I still see her and consider her to be a friend. My joints are increasingly tight and the legs and calves cramping. My neck is tight and upper back knotted. What a mess! She has her work cut out for her, but she is so sweet and so accommodating and makes me feel very comfortable.

I remain on the sleeping pills as I can only sleep with them. I have tried to ween myself off but can't sleep without them. I have become dependent on these but all my physicians are not surprised and stress the need for sleep.

August 7th - I have been looking for Biafine cream for my chest as I prepare for radiation. The hospital suggests it since your skin can burn and become tight. Brant Arts appears to be the only pharmacy who can order it for me. I go to Buffalo shopping with my friend Wendy and her daughter Sarah in hopes of finding this Biafine cream.

The weddings, Nat leaving to return to Ottawa for school and Bob being busy at his 3 basketball camps were too much for me to handle. I was overwhelmed and wanted this treatment and the way I have been feeling to end. Feeling alone.

August 8th - was Bob's birthday but we did nothing. Too tired I guess.

Even though I was thrilled to have completed my last chemo treatment on July 15th, I was exhausted, weak and emotionally drained. It took everything just get up and out of the house. Though I was aware that my radiation treatments were going to begin soon, I was too exhausted to worry.

Approaching Sunrise

CHAPTER 6

RADIATION

The day for my radiation treatments came quickly and my exhaustion kept me from worrying too much. Also, I thought the radiation treatments were going to be a "piece of cake". Little did I know that this was certainly **NOT** the case.

August 10ᵗʰ - RADIATION DAY. I go to the radiation clinic at 10:30 am and have no idea what to expect. I am going by myself as I work Mondays and the Juravinski clinic is 10 minutes from my work. I will try to plan my treatments at lunch so I do not disrupt my work and do my radiation at lunch. I don't know much about radiation but I have read the books and pamphlets in the waiting areas of the hospital. They say very little and I recall my Mom having no problems years ago with her radiation treatment.

I arrive early and wait a few minutes until I am greeted by a technician. She (Colleen) explains the process. She told me that they work as a pair so she was only one of my technicians. There are 4 technicians in this clinic and that there are many different clinics here at the cancer centre. Others in the waiting room appear to be different cancers, ages, sizes, everything... Some have people with them and some don't. They explain I will always have 2 of the 4 technicians for consistency and comfort. Today will be 40-50 minutes - the first one is longer to explain things and take pictures – but that in the future I should be 25-30 minutes. They advise me not to bathe as long and as much and keep my breast covered so it becomes less dry.

August 11ᵗʰ - I am in the next day at 11 am to receive my radiation. They have accommodated me around my lunch hours as I had hoped. I have the same two females (Team A) and feel more at ease as I know what to expect. It was frightening yesterday as I was uncertain as to what was happening. The radiation machine is big and scary. You are naked with a cotton robe and laying on this cold metal sheet with this huge piece of equipment over and beside you. It moves as they control it and you must stay still and it ZAPS you with radiation. A light beams on the area and you are facing a wall that says something serious like RADIATION TAKING PLACE – BEWARE!

The picture below is where I had my radiation treatments. The size of the machine freaked me out, as did the "High Voltage" and "Danger" signs surrounding me. The teams who supported me during these treatments were amazing.

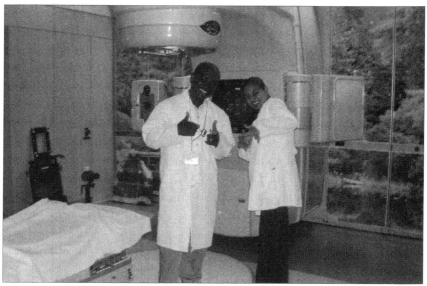

A picture of Team B just prior to the start of my treatment.

August 11ᵗʰ continued… Today was 25 minutes and I returned to work and worked until 5 pm, a full day. My Mom's birthday is tomorrow, August 12ᵗʰ, and we are going downtown to dinner to celebrate. We will go early as I get tired and am in bed by 7- 8 pm most nights.

August 12ᵗʰ - I meet the B team at radiation today; Michael and one of the other ladies from yesterday. They take much longer to get me ready as they are different together. The spots to radiate have to be spot on so I want them

A p p r o a c h i n g   S u n r i s e

to take the time to do it properly. My Mom is 77 today! We have a lovely dinner in downtown Burlington, including cocktails and wine. Perhaps I will sleep better when mixed with my meds. I am still taking 2 of my little blue pills to sleep. I call them my magic pills as I sleep well with them.

August 13th - (Day 4 of Radiation) - My right arm is so sore, as is my chest, shoulder and ribs. They ache and are tight. I have to place my right arm up above my head while the 6 beams of radiation hit me. It is uncomfortable and I am tense.

Another busy 9-4 day at work. Real busy, but it makes my day go by fast and I don't think of my aches and pains. Very therapeutic I think. My therapist Kim saw me again today and had to work on my right side and my neck as it was tight from the radiation. I was sad today and she saw it the minute she laid eyes on me. She feels my pain and sadness I think. Kim makes me feel better and is gentle but effective at the same time.

August 14th - I get the B Team again at the clinic. I tell them how sore and miserable I am. The evenings are very uncomfortable and I ache terribly. They explain the radiation is localized and should only tighten the area being hit, so they feel the other pain is a side effect of the Taxol chemo treatments.

My parents had friends visiting from Chicago so we entertained at our home. Why? I never want to cook, especially feeling as I do. I think they wanted to see the new house. Natalie surprised me with a gorgeous vase of flowers as she knew I was struggling - especially without her. That made my day!

Had a few cocktails and wine and took my sleeping pills. What a mess I was and I couldn't even sleep! I think I should lay off the alcohol as they suggest at the hospital when in treatment.

The weekend was organizing, shopping and running errands. I went to Port Credit to visit Paula – she has a new home too and I wanted to see it. Had a nice visit but so tired and was in bed early both nights. What fun I am!

August 17th - Here we go again. Same routine: work, radiation and home to bed early. Feeling exhausted, especially after the weekend and as radiation progresses. Getting to work just after 9 am since I get up about 7 and do my stretching and moving to get ready for the day. The A team today at radiation – my favourite two ladies who get me in and out quicker.

B team on Tuesday, then the same old day except only worked until 3 as I was tired. A Team on Wednesday but they struggled to get me in the exact perfect positions for some reason. This annoys me as I worry they don't get the right area to be radiated. Very tired lately and getting tired of this daily lunch routine. It is my brother Michael's 47th birthday tomorrow but he is celebrating in North Carolina where he lives with his family.

I do not have much to write as it's the same old thing; I am so miserable and my chest is tight and burnt. I have a darker skin tone and have never burned even when vacationing in the Caribbean or Florida. I am using the Biafine but it doesn't appear to be doing anything as I am red and getting tighter and more burned at each session.

I write nothing from August 20th–27th in my journal - I am unhappy and miserable and decide it is best not to write anything. What do they say, "If you can't say anything nice, say nothing."

Behind in my unpacking of boxes and still sorting through boxes. Feeling very unorganized and unsettled.

September 4th - Only two weeks of radiation left. My skin is so dark in colour and very tight. Feels tough like leather. I find radiation rough and prefer the chemo to this treatment. I have difficulty raising my right arm more and more each day. I do my exercises (the ones they showed me when I had the mastectomy) in the shower against the wall but it hurts more now with the radiation.

Post- Treatment Crash

All the books I read warned of a "crash" that can occur when an individual completes treatment. I ignored or skipped over those parts in the books because I did not think it would happen to me. But it did! This crash was the most paralyzing thing I ever went through.

CHAPTER 7

AFTER THE CRASH

A s thrilled as I was to be finished radiation and treatments at the Juravinski and say goodbye to all the support staff, I felt so abandoned and alone. The books tell you this may happen but I thought there was no way would this happen to me, especially given I had done so well. I could not get out of bed, I was numb and didn't care to do anything or go anywhere. I think this is how you feel when you have the "baby blues" or postpartum depression.

This MASSIVE sadness and feeling of not caring about anything or anyone just took over and HIT me so suddenly. I called Dr. Tozer and he said this was normal, then referred me to the Cancer Care Social Worker. He, and others, had said they couldn't believe how well I did from diagnosis to this point without a break or time off. I thought they were just being kind and making me feel good. I had been told I could take time and should not push myself, but never did I feel I was overdoing it!

Since I didn't acknowledge this transition time as perhaps being a difficult one, I hadn't given it any thought or preparation. My GP and Linda, my social worker, suggested antidepressants and a leave from work. I had only ever taken a few days here and there around chemo and a week after the mastectomy, so I listened and took their advice and took time off.

They explained (I also got this info from books and others) the effect this cancer and the chemotherapy and radiation (both aggressive) has on a body and our mental state. They assured me I wasn't crazy, even though I felt it, and they told me I have no control of this, which was frustrating. I was tired. I cried. More being tired. More crying. Didn't get dressed and just wished to be alone. This WAS NOT ME!

The social workers (I saw another one other than Linda) felt I had carried on for 9 months with such strength and courage trying to "keep it all together", that I didn't take the time for myself. I thought I had.

They suggested therapy, mental and physical, the wellness centres, a vacation and rest. I called Wellsprings in Oakville as Wellwood in Hamilton wasn't offering the Reiki and tai chi I was interested in.

As I was leaving my last radiation appointment, (get ready for another 'right time for something to happen' moment...) I bumped into Cheryl - an old friend I knew from Burlington from when our boys had played hockey and lacrosse together. We catch up and of course ask one another, "What are you doing here?" Perhaps dumb questions, especially since I have a cancer cap on, no eyebrows or lashes. Anyway, we discover we both are patients and she is just beginning her chemo.

We speak for a while, hug and discover we have both moved to the Carlisle area and are 2 Concessions away from one another – crazy! We agree to go together to the Wellness Centre and attend other seminars and programs that will help us! I am thrilled we ran into one another as everyone needs a "cancer buddy"! And we live 5 minutes away from one another.

How special to reconnect with someone from the past and share part of this journey. If we hadn't been in the right place in the hospital at the time we were, we would have never have been reunited at such a significant time in our lives. (The big guy is looking out for us. Or is it the angels I refer to in the beginning of this book?)

I am delighted about Cheryl, especially as I am home in this FUNK.

October 6th - is Saturday and it is the Breast Cancer run. I am part of Bev's team: BJ's Cuties. We raise enough money to place 3rd in the community teams. Family participated as did Isabelle, my friend and roommate from the hospital, and her family!

What an amazing group and all connected by our cancers. Not a bad thing! They say it takes a VILLAGE and this was our village team, walking and running together and sharing our survival and our commitment to the research and cancer causes. What an amazing day. I love all the photos despite my short grey hair growing in. It was made even more special when Nat's good friend Jen opened the ceremonies by singing "The Climb", the Miley Cyrus song (I mentioned it earlier in the book) that my friend Suzanne referred to in the care journal.

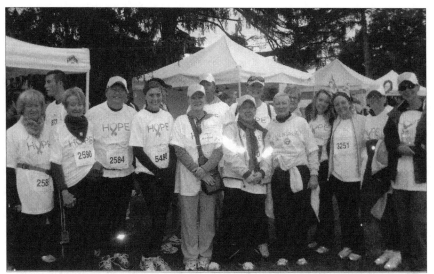

A picture of the team my friend Bev organized for the Run For A Cure.

"I can almost see it. That dream I'm dreaming but, there's a voice inside my head saying, you'll never reach it. Every step I'm taking, every move I make feels lost with no direction. My faith is shaking. But I gotta keep trying, gotta keep my head held high. There's always gonna be another mountain. I'm always going to want to make it move. Always going to be an uphill battle. Sometimes I'm going to have to lose.

Ain't about how fast I get there, ain't about what's waiting on the other side. It's the climb. The struggle I'm facing. The chances I'm taking, sometimes may knock me down, but, no I'm not breaking. I may not know where. But these are the moments that I'm going to remember most. Just got to keep going and I, I got to be strong, just keep pushing on. There's always going to be another mountain. I'm always going to want to make it move. Always going to be an uphill battle. Sometimes I'm going to have to lose. Ain't about how fast I get there, ain't about what's waiting on the other side, IT'S THE CLIMB".

When Jen sang this, there wasn't a dry eye in our group and many other groups watching her! This group of thousands were all touched by cancer and what a sight to see, a sight of love, support and HOPE! So Powerful and Encouraging! Hopeful and Empowering!

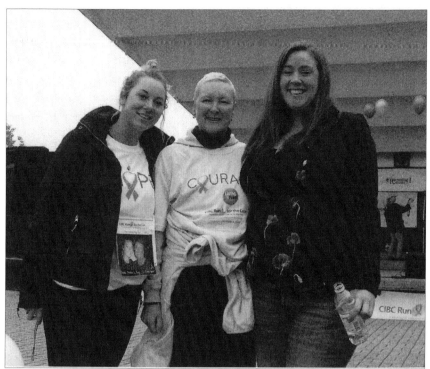
Natalie, me, and Jen at the event.

October 8ᵗʰ - I started my anti-depressants, just 30 mgs of Cymbalta. It also helps with joint pain so I get a 2-in 1 medication to help my head and my joint pain. Bonus! Next appointment with social worker, October 14ᵗʰ to follow up.

The week after the run I am also busy helping Brock organize his DRESS FOR EVERY BODY, fundraiser and fashion show for BC. I am modelling as are other BC survivors. He and Joelle are overseeing the fashion show, including the models and all the clothing!

October 24ᵗʰ - I write the last journal entry and want to stop the care site as I need to move on and not dwell on this.

My hot flashes are increasing as the treatments have thrown me into early menopause! Chemo does that and, sure enough, the flashes started soon into chemo. Stress and certain triggers set off the flashes, triggers like wine, coffee and chocolate, my 3 comfort items. Not fair! Heat and damp-ness are brutal and affect my joints terribly!

A DRESS FOR EVERY BODY

B rock Stacey has been personally touched by breast cancer as his mother is battling the disease. Brock, along with Teo Hair and Bodyworks and SB Prime Steakhouse hosted the 1st Annual Breast Cancer Survivor Celebration and Juravinski Cancer Centre fundraiser: A Dress for Every Body.

The night started out with a fashion show provided by Joelle's with models who have either conquered or are battling breast cancer. Very special musical guests were on hand to entertain. Amazing raffle prizes were donated including a beautiful Tiffany Keys Heart Key Charm necklace and a 6-day stay in Mont Tremblant. Congratulations Brock on an amazing event and good luck topping it next year!

Event by Alanna Jakubauskas

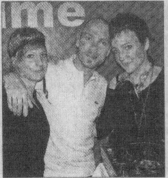

DJ Alicia Hush provided some beats

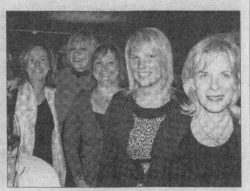

Karen, Margie, Deb, Katie and Heidi

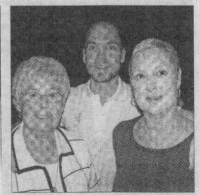

Brock - Event Coordinator with his grandmother Joan and his mother Joanne

My doctors agree to keep me on the sleeping pills as I have tried to ween myself off but can't and I need my sleep at this point in my healing. They suggest exercise, good diet and to continue with the meditation, yoga, Reiki, massage – whatever relaxes me and keeps me calm and not stressed. Dr. Tozer thanked me for my fundraising efforts at the Juravinski cancer centre - I had mentioned the activities in Burlington and my interest in becoming a member of the fundraising team at this cancer centre. I also volunteered to do peer support and to speak with others going through the same thing. I give my name to Wellsprings, Juravinski and my social workers.

The book AFTER BREAST CANCER is suggested by HesterHill Schnipper. I can't recall if I completed it. I gave so many books away and have a small library I have kept and purchased again for my own reference.

Dr. Tozer wants to discuss reconstruction in 6 months and says he would refer me to Dr. Avram.

October 24ᵗʰ – My last blog entry. It is time for this site to be over. It has been a long 10 months and I am tired. A friend said it is time for this breast cancer stuff to be gone and I agree. We have completed the run and had Brock's event so we are finished with the BC events for a bit.

It has been a journey I don't wish to take again and I hope none of you have to.

You have been an amazing strength and support and I could not have done this without you all.

We are blessed to have you all be a part of us and I will never be able to tell you what you did for me and my family. I said early in this journal that I needed all my angels and I wrote something like, "wrap your wings around my heart and heal me from my pain and fear".

You all wrapped me well and have helped me battle.

As many of you are aware, I have had to take a leave of absence from work as I am struggling with the depression and the side effects of the medications and treatments and am in a FUNK. It was too much – all that went on in my little body – this smaller, weaker body as I have lost much weight as some of you commented at the fashion show recently.

Speaking of the show, I have to say how proud I am of Brock, Emily and Shannon for their efforts and hosting an amazing SOLD OUT event this week. For your first event, you blew us all away and raised awareness and funds for the Juravinski cancer clinic.

So I leave this site with mixed emotions as it has been a huge support and got me through some of the toughest times especially in the beginning. Some of you have asked why I haven't written more – some days I couldn't as I was too tired or had nothing good to say and I was struggling!

It's a struggle I continue to fight and I will be patient and strong in the dark days.

At the event this past Thursday, I met some great women who have been through this and assure me this is all part of the process. I think the anti-depressants are starting to kick in and I am trying to wean myself of other medication. I am seeing people at the clinic who are helping me through this rough patch. I am doing all I need to do. I am hoping to start Tai Chai again and some meditation and will continue with my massage and Reiki. I need to find more energy to do these as I am really tired. These months took so much out of me. I felt better today so let's hope I am on the mend and able to return to a more normal routine. It has been an over-whelming time and I really feel I need this time to heal and rest. As you scroll through the site and the pics, I hope you take something from our journey together as it really has been one we all have learned from and will continue to learn and become stronger as a result. I look forward to seeing you all and speaking with you as we do and getting back to a different kind of normal after all this.

Love You
Joanne

October 28th – (*Dad's last comment*)....

> *Joanne, the tough times are almost over as we have all seen over the past weeks and with the success of the RUN and Brock's special night you are leaving this site on a high note. I have told you many times over the past weeks as we have spent more time taking care of one another, how day by day you were noticeably getting back to your old self even though you were still suffering from time to time. That is why I am writing this final note now. Typical of you, you wanted to look after me when mother was away following my surgery and I did enjoy our afternoon rest sessions which did us both good. From now on everything will only be good and you will*

get stronger and soon return to the full and active life we all love and admire you for. You just can't keep a great person down and you are one of them. You have the greatest bunch of friends that anyone could wish for and they will continue to be with you.
Your family are all very proud of you."

To see Dad have the last words on the Care site was nice and significant as my book and journey started with my parents, similar to the way Mom's journey began with me and Mom and Dad all together in Buffalo.

The month off was most valuable and much needed. It was a time of healing, discovery and recovery. I needed this time to review and regroup and understand what had happened to me over the past 9 months. My mind, body and spirit had taken a "shit kicking" and I didn't realize the impact it had on me and those around me. As they refer to it in books and how professionals speak of cancer survival, it is a NEW NORMAL. Now, how do you proceed? What is expected of me? What do I expect?

I am paralyzed mentally and physically but don't know why and I have no control. I can't snap out of this! I have always been a problem solver, a multi-tasker, stable and confident. What has happened to me?

I am so blessed to have many friends with me, especially Cheryl who is attending Wellsprings with me and hanging out with me. I have had lunch and outings with a few friends but I am not wanting to go out socially or be seen by others when I am depressed like this.

I have met some wonderful women in-patients and instructors at Wellsprings and at the cancer centre. They reinforced recovery and the need to heal and take this well-deserved time I needed. Recovery does become an important part of this journey. The sisterhood and comradery in these groups is comforting and powerful. The strength and courage found among some of the weakest and most vulnerable women we were surrounded with is so inspiring and life changing for me. We have turned our pain into empowerment!

We all need to take the time to reflect on all we have and what we are so grateful for. I have learned to recite and repeat my gratitude sayings and write in my journal, reaching out and sharing with others. In a short time I had others reaching out to me; part of my healing was to give back and share with them what I have experienced and learned.

To connect with strangers and to share something so meaningful and precious and become a part of them and their families is such a blessing and heals both of us. It is bizarre – and incredibly therapeutic - to get so intimate through our crises; I feel so fulfilled and blessed. We support and counsel one another and we educate each other in so much. We speak of our new diets, new skin care, our feelings, our fears, our families, our fight and our cancer!

As I became more educated and Lois encouraged me to look at my diet and skin care and what was more preventative and safe for me, I changed my food and skin care choices. I began staying away from harmful chemicals and phthalates and parabens and mineral oils which contribute to cancer and poor immune system, etc. I started sharing this with my BC buddies too as we all need to be better educated. I started attending the After BC workshops and seminars on nutrition and prevention - I wish more women would attend these.

My daughter Natalie had started educating me as she was eating healthier and was aware of the chemicals and nasty ingredients. She too has a curiosity as she has a great grandma, grandma and mom with cancer. She will have to go through the testing and we are told that she is at risk for it also. It took cancer to introduce me to a cleaner, safer way of life and that is great!

I also took a higher dose of Cymbalta, 100 mg. at this time.

I returned to work in early November and all was good. I slowly got back in the saddle! My colleagues are amazing and were the biggest supporters - I couldn't have done this without them.

I hated the short grey hair but you are advised not to color it for a while and when you do, it must be healthy, organic product. I have changed all my skin and hair care to chemical free, fragrance free, animal free, gluten free, etc.

I have become a loyal Arbonne client and am using the nutrition line too; I am now aware of the benefits of the protein shakes, detox items, etc. I do suggest these products but I mostly just want women and men to be aware of the ingredients in their products that may provoke or have a connection with cancer. Use any safer line and do your research. As a grandparent, I started using safer baby products so my grandchildren were brought up with safer, purer products. There are links to young children and cancer - especially boys and testicular cancer - that I became aware of, so please take note.

My next appointment with Dr Tozer is **April 12th, 2010**. Happy New Year!

Dr. Tozer is pleased with my progress. I have gained 10 lb since November 11th, 2009. He stressed the need for activity, good diet, weight gain and therapy for the joint and muscle pain. He stressed the need to return to work, recreation and my volunteer work, especially the work I find so rewarding at the cancer clinic. He was made aware of Brock's event, from which proceeds went to the Juravinski, and thanked me for my recent contributions with the fundraising committee of the cancer clinic he is very involved with. He believes we should consider reconstruction and will refer me to Dr. Avram. He was pleased with recent mammogram results and will see me in 6 months. He is ok that I remain on the sleeping pill since I struggle to sleep without them. He will reduce the anti-depressants (Cymbalta) to 75 mg and suggests I stay on them if there are no side effects. They help with joint pain too so I want to remain on them.

Dr. Tozer and team stress the need for: exercise, no tobacco, a good diet (prefer plant based), less sun exposure and to strengthen my immune system. Exercise has become one of the central components of cancer rehabilitation.

The next two pages outline my commitment to the awareness and treatment of breast cancer.

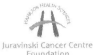

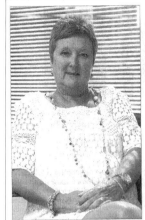

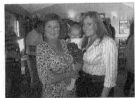

:: Joanne Stacey with her first grandbaby Rachel.

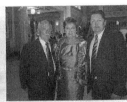

:: Joanne with her father and brother.

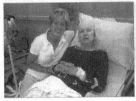

:: Joanne with her best friend Lois at chemo (she and her friend Kathy share in SNUGCAPS).

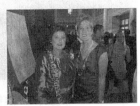

:: Joanne and Lois and two years after the chemo photo (left)—what a difference and reconstruction!

:: "I've taken control of my life. I surround myself with supportive people now. I don't sweat the small stuff anymore..."
— Joanne Stacey

Joanne Stacey

Hamilton woman's battle with illness gives her a brand new outlook on life.

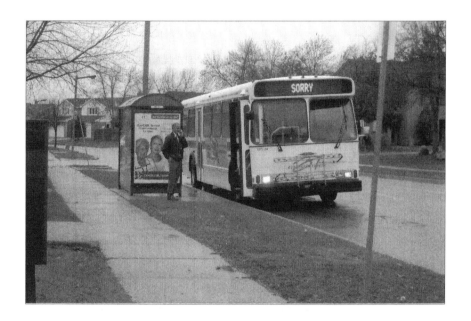

CHAPTER 8

RECONSTRUCTION

A s I mentioned in the beginning, I had never considered any further surgery after the mastectomy. A few friends had asked me to consider reconstruction at the same time as the mastectomy but everything moved so fast, and I was lucky to get a surgery date the week I was diagnosed, so my focus was on that surgery and just GETTING THE BREAST OFF AND THE CANCER OUT! Reconstruction was something I could consider later but at that time in February 2009 I wasn't ready.

The only thing I considered was having both breasts removed, something my surgeon advised me against. She explained the other breast is necessary as it would assist in detection of cancer again and told me to keep it. I gave it little thought as I trusted the surgeon. My only focus was to have my right breast removed and hope the cancer had not spread. I just wanted to be clear of cancer and on my way to healing. Others in the community spoke so well of Dr. Kancherla so I was not questioning anything.

The friend who asked me to consider the double mastectomy was the same friend who could not handle my cancer and just wanted me to feel as good as I could despite what was happening. I believe she thought a double breast removal would make me feel more normal. There was nothing normal in what was happening at that time. I know she wanted the best for me and also that she likes to plan and know all the issues to consider in order to make the best choices. However everything happened so quickly and we didn't have the time and luxury to know what would happen. I was blessed to have a diagnosis within a week and a surgery date in two weeks. That does not happen to most people, which is so unfortunate.

I mention this as you have to realize how this affects the people around you. Your close friends and family want the best for you but, at the same time, they are shocked with the diagnosis and want to take care of you or have some input into what should happen. You need to listen and let them speak their feelings as this is all part of your journey too! They are and will be a part of your life and you need them. You must acknowledge their worry and hurt and their fears. This is so important!

When I think back, I didn't listen enough to my daughter Natalie and how she felt leaving school and taking care of me. Some days I was short with her and I didn't recognize her worry and fears. My husband is another who I may have ignored as he just seemed so strong and was there for me in every way. Bob never said anything about reconstruction - he let me do my own research and make the decision. The one breast bothered me more than anyone else; I felt lopsided and the prosthetic was hot, heavy and so ugly! I had been away **in Florida** and carrying the prosthetic insert was inconvenient - the case is much like a hat case they give you when you purchase a lady's big hat. I always worried it was showing in my bathing suits even though my bathing suits were the special suits made for those who had an insert. It would just tuck in the flap of the right side where I had no real breast, much like the bras.

Fall 2010 - So, back to the reconstruction. Every time I looked in a mirror I saw the scars and no breast. I was reminded every day of the cancer. It was always there! I looked and felt unattractive and it was unnecessary as there were options to repair this and make me look more normal. I was disfigured, unbalanced and lopsided. Now it was bothering me so I wanted to look at the options and educate myself as to what the best option for me would be. The timing was right: I felt good about the cancer treatments and my radiation was over and I was healing well. I was back to work full time and all was well.

Bob never said anything about reconstruction but I know he prefers me to look more normal (have 2 breasts) and he supports whatever decision I make. I called Dr. Avram's office at the Hamilton General – this is the doctor I was given a referral to, and I had also heard about him through many of the cancer support resources and Julie at Greta's Flair.

I called that day as I was feeling courageous and felt very confident with this choice. Cindy in the office was so pleasant and was able to book me in within a few months. The waiting list was lengthy so I was fortunate to get in. I started to research the different procedures and forms of reconstruction and felt the tummy tuck/DIEP flap was my preference. Dr. Avram would suggest the best one but after all I had been through I thought a tummy tuck would be a great treat, despite how involved and painful the surgery may be.

Many of my friends encouraged me and were excited for me. They agreed that after a cancer diagnosis, mastectomy, chemotherapy, losing my hair, feeling so sick, radiation and the depression that followed, this was an exciting time for me and a tummy tuck was a nice gift to myself.

I was so excited to meet with Dr. Avram; his waiting list is very long so I was thrilled that this was going to happen sometime in the next year. The opportunity to look and feel more attractive and feel more desirable for Bob is amazing. His office assistant Cindy is so much fun and so encouraging that she made me feel even more at ease. I needed to feel that this was the right thing for me. Cindy took photos of my chest which was a bit awkward but I understood why they needed them.

We discussed the tummy tuck and specifically how the skin is raised to make the breast. He gave me options for a new nipple but we agreed to leave that as he knew of a tattoo artist who was tattooing nipples and he recommended her. A nipple was the least of my worries at this time. Dr. Avram was thorough and comforting and reassured me that this was the best procedure for me and I trusted him. I was thrilled that he was considering March 2011 for the surgery, specifically March 21st.

The anticipation was tremendous months before the surgery but I never second guessed myself and my decision. Before the surgery I had the mammogram and other blood work that I needed, then saw Dr. Avram on the morning of Monday, March 21st at Hamilton General. Bob took me in very early and we were in the pre-op area with other patients. I felt very relaxed and Bob sat with me until I was taken to the operating room. There were no issues, no waiting and we were so ready. I think Bob was worried as he knew the procedure was lengthy and I would be in the ICU afterwards, in great discomfort. Bob always remained strong for me and never showed his emotion, but I knew he worried and wished he could make things easier and less painful for me. He had seen me in enough pain the past years.

Being in the operating room never bothered me and I always looked forward to the anesthetic and counting and feeling high before being put to sleep. Best feeling ever!

I recall waking up very fuzzy and remembering the hallways and construction in the hospital as they wheeled me to my room in an ICU area. As confused and fuzzy as I was, I saw Bob with the nurses and saw a man somewhere around my bed. I realized quickly that I am in a coed ward with 2 other men and 1 woman. I am so uncomfortable that men are in my ward that I immediately tell Bob to do something!

I refuse to have a man across from me in this room considering I have had what I consider a fairly delicate surgery and my entire body is exposed - I am bandaged from chest to tummy and naked! Despite how groggy and sick I felt, I felt even more sick and uncomfortable with men in my room. Nurses were in and out and the drapes were open and I was so worried this man would see me naked. Bob tried to comfort me and told me he would ask why I was with men and would stay with me. I was sick and felt nauseous and was so out of sorts. Nurses were checking drains and monitoring things I wasn't really aware of. I just wanted to rest. I felt like I was tied up as the bandages were everywhere I looked. My throat was sore and a nurse explained I had a tube in my throat given the seriousness of the surgery. I didn't need to know that - before the surgery I had asked Dr. Avram to tell me little of the details since not knowing only makes me more anxious.

A team of doctors who work with Dr. Avram entered the room and I recall asking if there could be fewer people as I was feeling very sick and overwhelmed at that moment. They were very sensitive and I believe only a few remained in my room. The two best looking men remained and I felt I was in an episode of Grey's Anatomy.

Dr. Avram explained the surgery went well. I caught some of what he said about why nurses are checking on me each hour and that I would be attended to closely for the next little while. I was unable to move – I was throwing up and dry heaving so I needed Bob and my Dad to help me with a bowl. I wanted ginger ale as I felt it had helped in the past when I felt sick.

I recall little of the first night, but it turns out that I had some great nurses who had pinned my curtains and put a note on the curtain not to open the one that exposed me to the man across from me. The man beside me was very sensitive and the next day he apologized for the situation. He told me that he understood why I was uncomfortable with men in my room. The nurses were sensitive to this too – they advised me that they were hoping to move the men and have other women brought to the room. One good thing was that the man beside me was being discharged to another hospital and a woman was coming to join me as a roommate.

Day 1 - was rough and I was very sick. I either slept or threw up. My friend Alison who works at Hamilton General was very kind - she brought me the real ginger ale (Canada Dry) and held the bowl as I was sick.

My Dad came to visit and he took over from Alison - I needed help since I couldn't really move well. Everything felt tight and I didn't know what was what really. I had a catheter so I didn't have to walk to the bathroom. I had forgotten about that but, since I wasn't able to move, I was delighted.

Day 2 - Jamie and my granddaughter Rachel (4 months) came to visit and that made my day. I was starting to feel a little better and was able to eat some simple foods and drink. I was OK with my curtains being opened to see my female roommates and speak to other people. Anna and Cheryl were my first visitors and we had a few good laughs. It was so good to see them. Bob came every day as did my parents. Natalie was away at school and Brock did not like hospitals, so he stayed away.

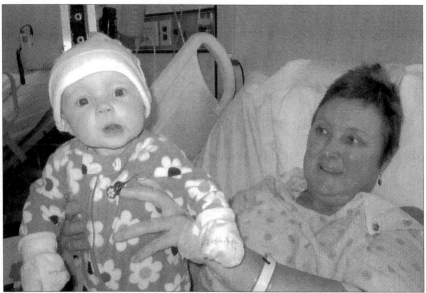

My beautiful granddaughter Rachel visiting me in the hospital.

Many friends called but it was a busy room and one patient had an infectious disease so we didn't encourage visitors. She was moved pretty quick; none of us felt comfortable as she was very sick and had some very unpleasant noises and movements coming from her bed area. I had a TV while many of the others didn't so I would turn it for them to see and turn the volume on. The bonding that happens with other patients is incredible and comforting.

Day 3 - They removed the catheter, so I was able to walk to the bathroom and wash and change into some real pajamas. This made me feel so much better. I started to understand what had happened in surgery, why my tummy was so tight and why the drains were in my chest and tummy. I felt good but didn't do too much other than rest and walk to and from the bathroom. I shared my skin care and lotions with my roomy next to me because she was off the streets and had no nice lotions. She was so appreciative and lovely despite her rough exterior. She had no place to live so she asked me for all my extra fruit and puddings to take when she was discharged. Very sad, and makes you realize how blessed we are to have all that we do.

Anna and Cheryl came by. It was so good to see them, despite how rough I still was and that I couldn't move too much. They had previously come before the catheter was removed when I was pretty quiet, hadn't washed and was still tired and recovering, so this was better timing. They bought me some lovely new pajamas and treats and we had a few good laughs! You have to keep a sense of humour, like I have through all of this!

Day 4 - A few more visitors. I was feeling much better and could get up and move around the room more easily, to the point that I was helping my other roommates when they needed it. I was able to wash my hair and body around the wounds and tummy and I started to feel like I was back to my old self with a new part. I was excited to see what this new boob would look like - and my tummy tuck! I had to be patient and knew I would see it all soon when the bandages come off and drains are out.

Bob came every day and was pleased to see me up and moving and feeling better. He can't believe how tough I have been through all these procedures. Mom and Dad were pleased to see me up and about and felt relieved that all seems to have gone well. The nurses were pleased with my progress and didn't need to monitor me as much, especially since I had fewer plugs on me. Was eating well and had good bowel movements, which is a must before one can leave hospital.

I was hoping to leave soon - I was doing well and was waiting for home-care to be arranged as part of the discharge plan. Enjoyed the days and evenings with visitors and watching television with my roommates (I still had the only television).

The girl beside me – the one who lived on the streets - was very appreciative of the TV and our friendship. She shared some very sad life stories with me. I saw the caseworkers and social services with her so I know they were true stories too. I really enjoyed her; it confirms that we must never judge and we can learn and take a little from all the people we meet, no matter how different they are. We all have something to share and she reminded me to be so grateful for all I have. It is easy to forget sometimes and feel entitled or take what we have for granted.

Day 5 – Dr. Avram and nurses were planning for my release as CCAC was in place and I was doing well despite how rough and sore my body parts were. I could recover in my own home and get the care from the nurses who would come to the house to check the drains and the tummy. The sutures were tight and I felt them always. I walk funny and can't bathe until the sutures and bandages removed.

I was discharged late afternoon and must share this story. Jeanne, the friend I have referred to throughout the story who has not dealt well with MY cancer and MY journey, planned to visit Friday afternoon - earlier that day my family told her I hadn't been released yet. Jeanne arrived at Hamilton General and asked reception for my room number. The receptionist said, "Mrs. Stacey is no longer with us." I had just been discharged so that is what the computer read. Jeanne refused to believe this as she had just spoken to my daughter Natalie and was told I was there in the hospital. Jeanne called Bob and couldn't reach him and started to panic - she thought something may have happened as I haven't spoken to her in 2 days. Jeanne was beside herself and asked the receptionist to clarify what she meant and again she was told, "She is no longer with us".

Jeanne continued to argue and asked if I had been moved to another facility or what is going on. Jeanne got hold of Natalie at work, saying it is urgent and that I am not in the hospital. Finally the two of them got hold of someone who knew I was on my way home.

Jeanne arrived at the house with flowers and shared this crazy story and the worry she felt as she thought I had passed. Why would a receptionist choose those words in a hospital setting? Why not say the patient was discharged? We recall this story and share it with many - this could only happen to my friend Jeanne.

I spent the weekend at home and had more guests visiting at the house. I lay fairly still on couch watching TV and visiting with friends and family. Great to be home and feeling well. Nurses great and drains out within a few days and sutures soon. Hope to go to work when the sutures are removed.

Nurse has taken bandages off and boob looks great and firm. Looks like a firm tight breast of a 14-year-old. I have no nipple yet but Dr. Avram and I plan to use the tattooist in Peterborough. The breast looks odd with no nipple but doesn't bother me. This breast is higher than my left but Dr. Avram will do a lift of that one later on. If I wore a good bra, they will look and feel level.

Next week the 140 sutures were removed by the nurse with her little suture kit she ordered. I felt every one pinch and felt the soreness and red that will be there after these are all pulled out. OUCH! She advised me of the creams to use on the incision and to watch for infection or any issues. Immediately, I felt less tight and free to move easier.

Plan to return to work on April 4th with tummy tuck and new right breast. Pretty excited!

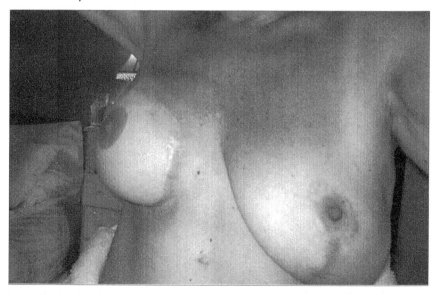

CHAPTER 9

POST TUMMY TUCK AND NEW OUTLOOK

I return to work in April 2011 and am feeling pretty good - and especially more attractive and HOT ! I have lost weight (presently 115) and lost my tummy. I also have 2 boobs and my new right breast is like the perky high breast I had in grade 8. Feeling pretty confident too!

My first week back at work I receive a warm welcome and many looks and questions. I don't know what people thought I would look like since it was just a replacement. I now look normal with 2 breasts of the same size. I wore the same clothes I always did and didn't change a thing. My hair was back and now colored so I was looking like I did before the mastectomy and now the reconstruction.

The only difference is that friends, colleagues and clients now see me healed - my outward appearance is as it was before the cancer diagnosis. When I had the mastectomy and returned to work, I always felt there was an elephant in the room. It seemed like I was treated with kid gloves; they worried about me having just one breast and didn't know how this may affect me. They didn't know where to look so I always wore my prosthetic or a scarf around my chest or a sweater or blouse that was loose so it brought little attention to my chest.

After the mastectomy, I was weak, bald, thinner, drawn and didn't have the energy I did before I entered chemo and radiation. They saw that and didn't know what to say or do. I attended a meeting at work with all the Directors around the board table a week after my mastectomy and I felt the discomfort, so, given the "ballsy" lady I am, I said let's just deal with this now. I pulled up my sweater and they saw all the bandages around my chest where my breast was and, as shocked as they were, it made us laugh and cleared the air. I had to let them know it was OK and I was OK. I wanted them to know I wasn't defined by a breast. For me, losing a breast was just a simple removal of a cancer; a disease I had to get rid of to survive. There was no other choice and in time I will decide on reconstruction or prosthetic or whatever. They also needed to see I am still the funny and real girl who can laugh and share.

This group was very important to me and were a huge support and are my extended family. I lost a breast, not my sense of self or humour or my spirit! I told them my treatment plan, what we can all expect and how, if at all, it may affect them if I am absent at times. I made them aware of my chemo dates and explained that I chose Wednesdays because I had Fridays off and could work Thursday and be back by Monday after being sick over the weekend. I felt they had to know that much would remain the same - I have learned that is what people worry about. Jon, my boss and very good friend, has been so supportive and sensitive, always accommodating me and always patient and reasonable.

All my other colleagues were amazing - they got me through so many tough days after chemo, asking me how I was on the days they could see my discomfort and joint pain. They recognized my fatigue and lack of energy at times, telling me they thought I was working too much and trying to keep up the same speed and routine. They know me well and knew I that I both needed to keep working and needed their support and understanding about it all. Like any patient, you want to return to the life you had before and keep things as normal as they once were - despite this NEW NORMAL everyone refers to. This always makes you feel safe and taken care of. Of course I was no different.

The summer was good and I decided to have my nipple tattooed on as Dr. Avram had suggested. I was ready to have real a nipple on my new breast, feeling that I looked silly without one. I was asked to try this new tattooist who specializes in breasts and faces and assisting women with facial or skin repairs. This is becoming a popular option for women because some surgeons prefer not to do a nipple. Dr. Avram would have, but at the time I was just focused on the surgery. I did my research and decided to try her: she was up north and we had friends in the area we could visit so Bob and I made a weekend trip of it. It was about a 2-hour tattoo session and was like any other tattoo. She asked me to choose size and colour so we could match it to the other breast. I liked her and trusted her. She explained it would scab like any tattoo but after the scab came off it would take the color and appearance of a real nipple.

I was impatient to see how it would look but she said it would be a few weeks before it looked good. My tattoo started to get dry and scabbed and as it peeled off the coloring of the tattoo did too, leaving it faded and looking nothing like it was supposed to. I was disappointed and took pictures of it to send to her.

My friend Barb, from work, took the photo as I sat across from her desk - we laughed as we shut the blinds to her office and thought how no one would believe what we were doing. It felt like a porno photo shoot, similar to when Dr. Avram's nurse took the pics of the breasts before surgery. After you have showed so many people your breasts and been exposed during surgeries, you don't really care who sees your lady parts anymore.

The tattooist and Dr. Avram agreed this nipple was not right: she agreed to redo it but I had no interest since they only stay on your breast for 6-8 months anyways. Makes no sense to me. I decided on the stick-on nipples Julie from Greta's Flair suggested and they were fabulous! We matched to the colour and size of my left nipple and all was great. I surprised Bob with them on vacation and he had a good laugh. You get 2 in a case, and a cleaning solution, for $50 dollars. Perfect! After this type of surgery you definitely want a nipple - nothing looks odder than one nipple through your bra especially in a T-shirt! You ladies know what I am talking about.

Life went on and the only thing bothering me was my tummy; the 140 sutures from the tummy tuck were still tight and I would feel the pull at times when I forgot. The scar is ugly but is so low that Bob and I are the only ones who see it.

I continued to work and live as I did before but busier. I did more Reiki, wellness programs and attended massage, meditation and other more holistic and relaxing techniques - this was all a part of my healing and exercise for the body and mind. I became more involved with the Wellsprings and Juravinski Cancer Centre peer support programs and became friends with others during their journeys.

I became a member of the fundraising committee at the cancer centre. I had a passion for this work: I wanted to give back beyond participating in the local RUNS and community events. These events were therapeutic and healing for so many reasons. We are not only giving back - we are surrounded by survivors and families of survivors, helping those who may have lost someone and being there for them tell their story.

I attended the DRAGON BOAT RACING Club as I thought that would be good for me. I learned quickly that I was not ready. These women are warriors, often much older than me and in better shape. I enjoyed the comradery but could not do the physical work. I was so inspired and blown away by these women, women of all shapes and sizes, ages and backgrounds.

The courage and commitment and way they overcame their physical challenges was inspiring and unbelievable. I didn't have their energy and the grit to do this - I was OK with that as I was still weak, without strength or mobility in my right side, and felt so out of shape. They took this Dragon racing seriously - they were dedicated and committed to the upcoming events and made it clear they had no room for weak links. I got to know some fabulous ladies and survivors; some who quit because they were still healing or had their cancer return, but all warriors and amazing women.

Sometime in the middle of 2011, Lois, Kathy and I shared the desire to do something for the Breast Cancer community. We had a few dinners and lunches with wine and laughs, and I came up with the idea of making comfortable cotton chemo caps. I had to purchase mine in the US (in Dallas) and have them shipped to me and it seemed liked there must be a better way. I gave several of mine away but kept a few of my favourites just in case I need them again. (There is always that thought of cancer returning.) I could also use these in the winter or around the house on a bad hair day.

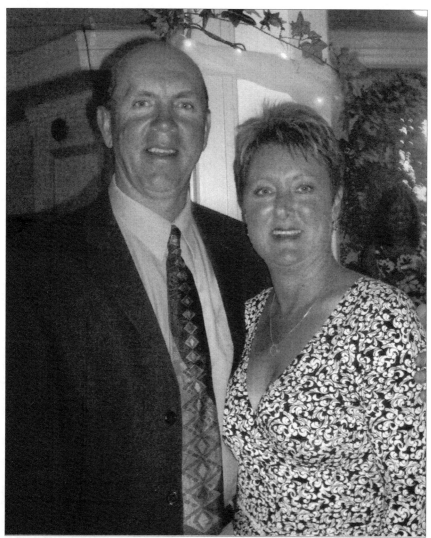

My husband Bob was my ROCK throughout this journey.

After much thought, research and travelling to many stores and hospitals, we agreed there was a need for inexpensive and soft head covers. SNUGCAPS was born. Lois was the Administrator, Kathy was the designer and sewer and I was the marketing person. We had always wanted to be in business together so here was something simple, not too expensive and, most importantly, needed – especially when we saw what was out there and how expensive they were. Despite our $1000 each start-up costs, our quick few sales at the clinics I was involved with and a few hospitals and stores and pharmacies purchasing some, we closed the business a year later and donated most of the caps.

We enjoyed spending more time together and making our caps but we didn't receive the interest we thought we might, and didn't get the support of the cancer clinics. In the end, we sold them off at our cost to those friends and families who knew patients or took some just to be nice. We felt good about the donations to the clinics and Wellsprings.

I sold a few to a running group as they thought some of them were great for the running especially in the cooler weather. We had fun and really didn't have the time it would take to make more and market our caps but we tried. This was a feel good hobby not a money making business and that was OK!

CHAPTER 10

LIFE LESSONS LEARNED

Turn lemons into lemonade. Put a different, positive spin on it. I realize I was - and am - blessed to have met the other women whom I now have strong relationships with. We are a sisterhood of women and families who shared fears, pain, and our courage. I met some of the most amazing women who I share a special bond and understanding.

And I got a tummy tuck out of it all! This is one of the perks, and definitely so is having no more periods!

Don't sweat the SMALL stuff! Cancer has made me realize how life is so precious. We must not waste time on the silly, petty STUFF. Worry about what really matters - life is too short!

Embrace the bald. I took control the day I knew it was a matter of time before the side-effects would have all the control and all my hair would fall out. Shave your head: make the decision to remove your hair before the chemo and cancer does. How fun to be bald and try different hair styles and colors. You won't get that chance again. I lost my hair in the summer, a hot and humid summer so being bald was powerful and so comfortable.

Remain genuine and real. Be honest with your feelings and those of others. What growth will occur? Your true authentic self needs to be reached and you will be stronger for it in so many ways!

Be blessed to be surrounded with such support – family and friends. I was so fortunate to have the professional team so close at the Juravinski to care for us and our community.

Preparation for anything. What is your Plan B? Are you ready for a crisis? How do you deal with a crisis?

How did you show your children and friends to deal with this? What have you taught them and shared together. What a valuable lesson they have been a part of!

NO MORE PINK or Pink ribbon tattoos! Everyone bought me pink - the BC color. At the time I was appreciative of the pink stationery, journals, socks, etc. but it got to be too much. I own every BC item available, even pink BC dog collars and leashes! Pink sweaters, pink underwear, socks with the cancer logo, and it goes on and on. I wanted something to remain with me from this experience, but none of the Pink "STUFF". Instead I got a martini/cocktail glass tattoo on my foot to symbolize fun and girlfriends!

Natalie and I went to my parents' home in West Palm Beach and we decided to do it there. It was an impulsive 'want' but I have learned not to plan everything and enjoy doing something crazy!

I now have no FEAR of dying and became more spiritual. It opened me up to so much I would have not experienced if I hadn't ever been diagnosed.

I can help others - something I have always tried to do my entire life - but now my path and passion is clearer and more focused. I was always involved with Breast Cancer awareness but I became more involved as I shared my experiences and story. I am a better resource and have offered my services to all the services I participated in. I launched my modeling career with Brock and Joelle's events! I did something I thought I would never do and did it well while raising money for the charities. What a feel good! It doesn't get any better than that!

I never thought I would write a book – wow! I am an author and I have the ability to help so many with this book. Proceeds will go directly to Juravinski, Jo Brant, Wellsprings and the Nanny Angel Network.

I learned to say NO and let others do my work and help me. To be vulnerable and let people cook my meals, drive me to chemo, clean my house, was HUGE for me. I also lost control and this is something every-one should experience. It is OK to break down and give in. My crash after the radiation was the best healing ever and I wish others would take this time.

It allowed me time with my Mom and Dad. I took the time off when my Mom was not well and that is the most important. I retired last year when I knew the book needed to be completed so that Mom could see it finished. She is a big part of this and will always live on through it. I hope she makes the first book launch. Stay tuned to hear if she does.

I must share something that needs to be stressed as a LESSON LEARNED and a part of this amazing SISTERHOOD, so this is the perfect place in the book to write about it!

Call it fate, destiny, divine intervention, a magical coincidence or SERENDIPITOUS!

Call it AMAZING! This is how I feel about all the unexplained events and people that were in my life before the diagnosis and returned during the journey and guided and supported me on this path. Call them my Lois, my Isabelle, my Jeanne, my JoAnne, my Cheryl. Call them inspiring, so much so that I have to compare them to the girls in the "SISTERHOOD of the TRAVELLING PANTS". Many of you have had a good cry when watching one of these 2 films. If you recall, the jeans held the MAGIC of keeping them close. The pants saw them through hardships, love, death, crisis, loss, celebrations and times of CHANGE!

A quote from the film states, "I think the pants got lost on purpose. That was their gift to us. They brought us back together. Back to a place of love, forgiveness and an understanding that what we have shared was all the magic we could ever need." What I love is how this quote connects to my book. The girls are in a boat watching the sunrise. Their story, as this one does, ends with the beautiful colour of the sun and says, "…moments of summer, looking out at the blending of the sea and sky, I realized it was a colour I knew very well, the softly faded essential blue of a well-worn pair of pants. The pants had brought us together again. The rest is now in our hands".

My ending is in my hands too and defeating this cancer was my doing.

That is a perfect summary of how I feel my cancer was. The gift that reunited us and involved many more back into my life and more closer to me. As Fran Drescher put forth, it is the most beautiful gifts that come in the ugliest and unpredictable packages!

The most incredible was reconnecting with Cheryl after 20 years and sharing our cancer battle. The other was Lois choosing to visit me as my mastectomy bandages were being removed, leading to Lois and I unknowingly being under the #5 Lifeguard booth on Clearwater Beach on my birthday, 5 years after survival. How precious and magical! Always **believe** in those magical moments.

Sisterhood and Education

Much of 2010 – 2014 was fairly normal or shall I say my NEW NORMAL as it is referred to. An unexpected, and very healing, element was the girl-friends I made and everything that we shared on our journeys. Taking part with the Reiki and Tai Chai at Wellsprings with Cheryl opened me up to a new group; a group of very vulnerable but strong women wishing to heal and having the courage to put themselves out there with others.

Some women become more isolated and can't be around others, not seeking out the support and resources available. I cannot stress enough the support and love I received from these groups and still do. Some relation-ships are more intense than others, some women are more ill than others and some friends you lose. I have lost 3 amazing women who fought a most courageous fight and taught me so much. What is so hard is that you become attached to their families while you are all sharing the same fears and struggles.

We were able to confide in one another, to laugh and to cry, knowing it was all ok and part of the healing process. No one can and should go this alone! I met women who did go it alone – not having a choice since they didn't have friends and family here. Can you imagine how lonely and frightening that is? It's like the seniors in a hospital who have no family and get no visitors or attention while in a ward and watching others get visits and family care.

I also started speaking more to my friends and colleagues about my cancer and treatments and prevention. Often people are not educated for many reasons. They are afraid to hear about it, it puts the possibility out there as something they might get or they just don't think it will ever happen to them. Do you know that a mammogram (x-rays of the breast) can detect 80 to 90% of breast cancers, even ones too tiny to be detected by a manual breast exam? This was me! Studies show that mammograms can cut the death rate of women in their 40's by 29% (Dr. Ox Swedish study).

While we are talking mammograms, I discovered that some women apply a topical painkiller (an OTC 4% lidocaine gel) to their breasts before their mammogram and experience much less pain. Two hours before your appointment apply the gel - no more than one ounce. Wash the gel thor-oughly an hour before the test as it can interfere with the image results. For women who have dense breasts or a family history of cancer, ultrasound is best to detect the abnormalities. I needed the ultrasound to better confirm my results.

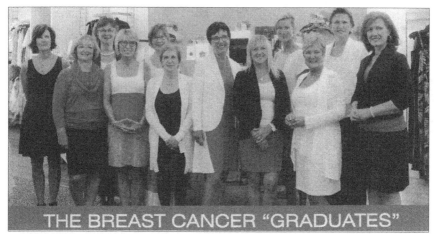

THE BREAST CANCER "GRADUATES"

This is a picture of my Sisters!

So getting back to my "survivor sisters" or graduates as we called ourselves recently at Joelle's last fundraising event (as we were getting tired of being referred to as survivors). These women bring an understanding and comfort you need while on this journey.

I have watched Robin Roberts (Good Morning America host), Kaley Cuoco (actress from Big Bang Theory), Diane London (former GMA host), Amy Robach (GMA news anchor) and many more go through this publicly. Perhaps most notably Angelina Jolie received great attention for her decision to have a double mastectomy, and in doing so raised awareness of the need for education. Those celebrities have a platform. I don't, so I have to write this book for all the women like me. This book is my platform and my way to educate, my way to have you share in my journey to help you and others.

As funny as it sounds, I feel connected to Robin Roberts and others who have shared their cancer story. I even wrote to the Good Morning America show in hopes of speaking about my cancer, and even join other women at a Breast Cancer awareness event at GMA.

My group of friends were the reason I could cope and be treated and heal well. Your cancer becomes a mental thing, and attitude and outlook contribute to healing and your after-cancer life and well-being.

My girlfriends and boyfriends, our kids' friends and acquaintances rallied for us! I say US because it was my entire family that was hurting and affected by this nasty disease. The kids are afraid their mom is going to die and the parents feel helpless and hate to see their child ill. They would take their place in a minute. Never assume how someone is feeling - everyone deals with it differently. I recall how thoughtful and helpful it was when a friend brought Bob a book about the husband's response.

I recall my Dad being so upset and so afraid, and all he could do was hope I was ready to fight. After all, you are the only one who can fight the fight and win. They can't do it for you! Brock, my eldest son was similar – he felt helpless and worried that I wouldn't do the treatment right, or wouldn't exercise or eat as I should and would not follow the doctor's follow up.

Many times I sensed their worry and feelings of helplessness despite how much I assured them I was ok and doing what I should. If they saw me having a few bad days, they felt I was weak and giving up. It was difficult to balance my illness and physical sickness (nausea, vomiting, and pain) with healing and a feeling of hope. Some days I did wish to be alone – at times I didn't know if I could be strong and "tough it out". Some days I wanted to give up and give in, but I didn't let most people know that. It is a real balancing act at times. Your friends, and others along the journey, get that. Remember that you can talk to them about it and be honest with them. They become your biggest resource and your biggest fans!

I have so many stories to share, some of which I have done already in this book, but one I must tell about is my Easter dinner in 2009. It was the weekend after chemotherapy, the days when I always felt rough. This weekend was really rough and I didn't want to think of dinner, of having to look at or prepare food - as weak and nauseous as I felt I just didn't care about anything. I stayed in bed the day prior and the day of Easter.

Without me aware of it, my good friend JoAnne prepared an entire turkey meal – with all the trimmings - and delivered it to our home just when the family was planning what to do for Easter dinner. It doesn't get any better than that! She, as were many others, was always there for me. Barb, my colleague at work, took her lunch hour to attend the chemo orientation with me and each day after that was there for me with a hug, a smile or an understanding of the day I was having – even taking her time to help me at work with simple tasks.

The stories go on and on about the people who became my angels and my strength that I depended on. Even crazy Jeanne, who finally came through after the shock of my diagnosis, was there every day with a good laugh, a treat or to tell me how sad she was and how she hoped this would go away. Her fears were great and we needed to discuss that. As she said, "this isn't just about you…. it's about me too." How honest and raw is that!?

I want to share something a friend sent me recently as the timing is perfect and fits here nicely.

"The women whom I love and admire for their strength and grace did not get that way because shit worked out. They got that way because shit went wrong, and they handled it. They handled it in a thousand different ways on a thousand different days, but they handled it. Those women are my super-heroes." Elizabeth Gilbert

This is so true, so powerful and so timely given what I am trying to say about these amazing women who touched my life, and will continue to do.

Tell the neighbor who tries to avoid you in the grocery store or by the driveway that it is OK not to know what to say. Tell them they can just say that they don't know what to say and they are here for you. That is enough. It is simple but lets the patient know you are struggling with it but there for them. It is more hurtful being ignored!

Allow your friends to deal with it as they must. Let them express how they feel and any discomfort or worry they may have. This is real life and real feelings. You will return the favour one day; already I have as some of my friends have been ill, or their parents were ill, and I did the same for them as they did for me!

It Takes a Village

This is so important and probably the most significant part of my healing. I have always been involved in my community and chose Breast Cancer as my charity of preference because I enjoyed working with Joelle and her many events and fundraising efforts. We made a good team!

After all my treatments, and after meeting many survivors and getting to know some of the Juravinski staff, I volunteered to sit on their fundraising committee where I helped organize the TEA for TWO. I still remain involved in the Gala I had been involved with through Investors Group when we were community partners.

Jon let me oversee the events, as he usually did, but for these, having been through this journey, I was more passionate and involved. I shared a stronger vision for the success of these events and I felt more of an ownership. I was now a model and participant in Joelle's fashion shows as we chose to have BC graduates be the models rather than hire models from a local agency. This was so well received and now I have had three modeling gigs!

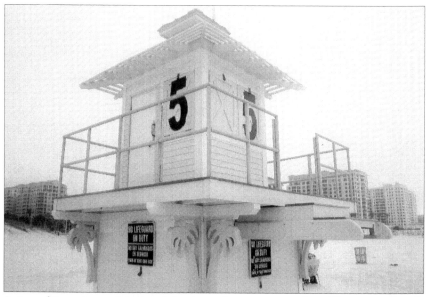

Lois and I went on a trip to celebrate my 5 years cancer-free. We sat on a beach and did not realize until later that behind us was this lifeguard tower #5! Lois and I now celebrate each February.

I am more committed than I have ever been in the prevention of and education about cancer. I have taken more of a personal interest in nutrition and caring for my body. I have changed all my skin care as I cannot use any harmful products with parabens and phthalates, substances directly linked to cancer. Mineral oil is another ingredient to stay away from.

The cosmetic industry is big business and they don't care about the effects their products may have. Our standards are the lowest in the world (along with the USA) and we need to be educated and aware. The Health and Environment Ministers have finally admitted we need to monitor the ingredients and standards and that there will be changes! My family and household uses new Arbonne products, which is safer for all of us. My pets also use healthier product and I have changed my housecleaning products too. It needs to become a safer way of life. Cancer is on the rise: now it is 1 in 3 women who will be diagnosed with some form of cancer. Children's cancer is growing too - testicular cancer in boys is an example which has been linked to harmful ingredients.

We all have a responsibility to raise our children in the healthiest possible environment - I didn't realize until 2009 that I was using unsafe products. I have taken the time to do my research and learn about nutrition and cosmetics. I am not saying my suggested products are the best – of course there are others out there - but do your research, take an interest in what you put on yourselves and your children and what you digest.

After treatments, your body takes a "shit kicking" and you need to get strong and healthy again to regain your physical health and mental state.

I am so proud of the work I have done and will continue to do in our community. We have an amazing one here, and I have shared this journey with my amazing TRIBE of beautiful people and good friends.

CHAPTER 11

SUNRISE

The book may be completed but the story goes on. I still have Mom here waiting to read the book despite her present struggles. I have many more women to help and I am more excited than ever that my efforts will reach many. I am more involved in all the community projects and am committed to improving the communication of resources and support services to all women.

I hope this book touches you in some way and provides some comfort and courage you may need. Cancer is not a death sentence - you can control the way you embrace it and take control and nurture your body, mind and spirit. You can influence others and provide the education and awareness we all need.

I must tell you that there IS a light at the end of the tunnel, a very bright light! To see the light and to get on the healthier, happier path it takes time, patience and HOPE! It takes belief to come out of the COLD and fear into the WARMTH and growth, much like nurturing a plant. You must nourish and nurture your body and spirit and work hard and not give up. As written in the biblical sense, and in many lyrics, light connects our BELIEFS. As Jon Jurus began the book with a quote, I will end with one:

> *"You will do well to pay attention to it, as to a light shining in a dark place, until the day dawns and the morning star rises in your hearts. Darkness will be dispelled and believers will walk in the purity, peace and joy in the light."* (2Peter1:19)

Living and sharing our story and working within our dark and light moments allows us our depth. I embraced that depth and have become a stronger, more courageous and passionate person.

The Light of the World is simply a Celebration of Life and today I celebrate my family, my sunrise!

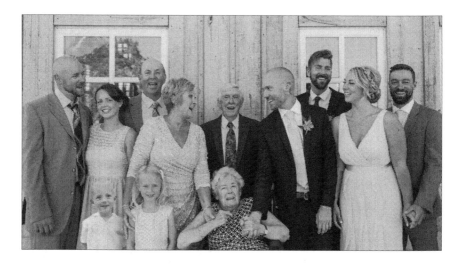

61472032R00072

Made in the USA
Charleston, SC
23 September 2016